Introduction to Intra-Operative and Surgical Radiography

Introduction to Intra-Operative and Surgical Radiography

JIM HUGHES

CT Radiographer
Leeds Teaching Hospitals NHS Trust
Leeds, UK

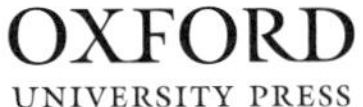

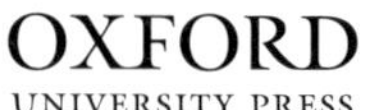

Great Clarendon Street, Oxford, OX2 6DP,
United Kingdom

Oxford University Press is a department of the University of Oxford. It furthers the University's objective of excellence in research, scholarship, and education by publishing worldwide. Oxford is a registered trade mark of Oxford University Press in the UK and in certain other countries

First Edition published in 2018

Impression: 1

Published in the United States of America by Oxford University Press
198 Madison Avenue, New York, NY 10016, United States of America

British Library Cataloguing in Publication Data

Data available

Library of Congress Control Number: 2018937421

ISBN 978–0–19–881317–0

Printed in Great Britain by
Bell & Bain Ltd., Glasgow

Endorsements

I welcome this well-written text to the world of medical imaging. There are many excellent aspects that will make it a useful addition to both university and clinical reading lists, and I especially praise its logical approach, excellent line diagrams, and use of page-corner icons to help the reader navigate content easily. The author uses a level of language suitable for academic use, yet it is easy to understand.

Undergraduate radiographers will benefit from the valuable underpinning that the text will provide before they attend theatre procedures for the first time, a vital start that will build confidence for the imaging newcomer in the surgical team. I also see benefits for those involved in clinical education, who wish to help with this introduction while developing mentorship skills.

There has been a long-standing need for a text of this type in the radiography profession, and I believe that this book will address the shortfalls in this subject area. I would like to congratulate the author on his excellent work.

Elizabeth Carver, formerly Deputy Director of Radiography, Lead for Clinical Education, Bangor University, UK (retired).

This is a well-written text, introducing the fundamental knowledge required to successfully perform common intra-operative imaging procedures. The concise review of equipment complements an overview of common surgical procedures that require imaging. The easy-to-follow descriptions, with the key projections required for each case, is supplemented by clear diagrams and images throughout. This guide will be extremely useful for student radiographers as well as newly qualified staff as they gain experience and competency in theatre imaging, and will be a handy reference for all radiology departments.

Nick Woznita, Clinical Academic Reporting Radiographer, Homerton University Hospital and Canterbury Christ Church University, UK

This an excellent book and a perfect guide for newly qualified radiographers who have been out of theatre practice for a while. I think this would be perfect to keep with the image intensifier as a guide, and can be used as a quick reference to advise the radiographer on how to operationally set up prior to a theatre case. The images of patient positioning are very informative, which again will aid the radiographer in the setting-up procedure for a theatre case. The examples of the images acquired from the image intensifier are useful in demonstrating to the radiographer what the surgeon will be expecting in terms of quality and the anatomy demonstrated on the image.

I would definitely be recommending that we purchase this book at my trust to provide more knowledge and information to our radiographers on theatre imaging.

Liza Field, Consultant Radiographer, Mid Yorkshire NHS Trust, UK

An informative and easy-to-read book that will be a useful tool for students and radiographers alike. Covers everything – from the inner workings of the image intensifier, to step-by-step guides for a wide range of operations.

Jamie Jordan, member of The Society of Radiographers, UK

Acknowledgements

This book would never have been possible without the support of my family, and also the resources and guidance from Emma Jones, Carole Burnett, the AO foundation, April Peake, Caroline Smith, Elizabeth Carver, and the radiology department of Leeds Teaching Hospitals NHS Trust.

Also thanks to Leah, my eternally patient partner, for her support and enthusiasm throughout.

Contents

Terms and abbreviations

AED	Automatic exposure device
ALARP	As low as reasonably practicable
AP	Anterioposterior
ASIS	Anterior superior iliac spine
Binning	The process of combining detector elements to increase sensitivity and reduce the amount of image data in a flat-panel system, at the cost of reducing spatial resolution
Collimator	A device for shaping X-ray beams using lead strips
CSF	Cerebrospinal fluid
CRIF	Closed reduction with internal fixation
DAP	Dose area product
DEL	Detector elements (the individual areas of the receptor in a flat-panel system)
DHS	Dynamic hip screw
DSA	Digital subtraction angiography
ESD	Entrance surface (or 'skin') dose
ESIN	Elastic stable intramedullary nail (a flexible intramedullary implant often used in paediatric long bones)
Ex fix	External fixator/fixation
EM	Extramedullary (outside the medullary canal of a bone)
FFD	Focus–film (receptor) distance
Flux	The amplification of an image through the input phosphor–photo cathode–output phosphor chain
FPD	Flat-panel detector
HBL	Horizontal beam lateral
II	Image intensifier
IM	Intramedullary (within the medullary canal of a bone)
IRMER	Ionizing Radiation (Medical Exposures) Regulations 2000
kV	Kilovolt
kVp	Kilovolt peak
LAO	Left anterior oblique

LIH	Last image hold
lp/mm	Line pairs per millimetre (the standard measuring system for spatial resolution)
mA	Milliamperes
Mag	Magnification
mAs	Milliamperes per second
Mb	Megabyte
Minification	The conversion of a large image into a smaller image
Noise	A random sequence of light and dark shades on an image that degrades image quality
OFD	Object–film (receptor) distance
ORIF	Open reduction with internal fixation
PACS	Picture archiving and communication system
Pb	Lead
Phosphor	A chemical substance that converts the energy striking it to light
Photocathode	A charged plate that releases electrons in response to light striking it
QA	Quality assurance
RAO	Right anterior oblique
Receptor	A system that receives an incidental X-ray beam and converts it to a visible image
Scatter	Radiation that is deflected away from the receptor by attenuating structures in the beam path
SIJ	Sacroiliac joint
SNR	Signal-to-noise ratio
TEN	Titanium elastic nail (a flexible intramedullary implant often used in paediatric long bones); see also 'ESIN'
THR	Total hip replacement
TKR	Total knee replacement
TSP	Trochanter stabilization plate

1

Introduction

Despite being one of the most common roles for radiographers, there is a dearth of available information on performing imaging during surgical procedures. Radiography practice (including theatre imaging) is often learned on-site at a teaching hospital, concluding with a practical assessment once students have gained enough experience. However, the long duration of many surgical procedures coupled with limited placement time prevents many students from experiencing as many procedures as they may like to. In addition, similar procedures may vary widely depending on the surgical requirements of each case. As such, this book is aimed at helping students and recently qualified radiographers in improving their knowledge and skills while not on theatre placement.

A full guide to every conceivable procedure that requires imaging would resemble a small library more than a guide book. As such, the more common procedures will be covered here in the most basic form. Every procedure can (and often will) vary from how it is described here, and so this book is neither intended to be a comprehensive guide nor a definitive one to imaging during procedures. It is aimed as a primer for those working in theatres as radiographers and as a quick reference guide for cases that one may be unfamiliar with. It is important to be able to adapt to events and restrictions during surgical cases, and this includes the production of good-quality and diagnostically effective images. If in doubt, the radiographer must discuss with the surgeon or the theatre team on what is required, and should never be afraid to ask for advice.

For those who may be looking for further information about surgical procedures, there is a wide range of literature available online. An excellent source of information is the AO foundation website, which covers orthopaedic procedures and techniques in great detail. Other sources are included in the recommended reading list for each section.

While working as radiographers in theatres, even though imaging is not taught as extensively as other areas of radiographic practice, there is no reason why we cannot improve our skills and experience in this area. It is our duty as professionals to ensure that we provide the best possible service while minimizing radiation doses to both the patients and theatre staff, including ourselves. Practice and experience are, of course, important in this respect; however, it is the opinion of the author that the practical knowledge should be shared widely to help improve professional skills.

Beyond professional competence, it should also be noted that interventional imaging in theatres is one of the most wide-ranging and fascinating areas of radiography, covering many specialties and innumerable procedures, all aimed at positive outcomes for the patient. Theatre imaging is different from so many areas of radiography as the radiographer is directly involved in the intervention and treatment of the patient, rather than just in the diagnosis and identification of pathology. It does not pose the question 'what is wrong with this person', but rather 'how can we fix it'. For centuries, surgery was a desperate and agonizing last attempt to aid people where other techniques had failed, but today it is an everyday miracle, a routine event that is the result of endless scientific advances in innumerable scientific disciplines, resulting in techniques and procedures that have massively improved the lives of millions who would otherwise have suffered or died from their ailments. Safe and effective surgical intervention has been one of the greatest achievements in medicine, and it is both an honour and a privilege to be involved in this complex and fascinating arena of healthcare.

Finally, kindly make note that the term 'theatre' is often used in this book to indicate the room where surgical procedures take place. This term is widely used in the UK; however, the term is also synonymous with other descriptors such as 'operating room' and 'surgery'.

2

C-arm systems

The need for a method to perform real-time X-ray imaging during surgical procedures led to the development of C-arm and mobile C-arm imaging systems, which have the ability to perform real-time motion or cine imaging series as well as still images. Fixed larger units are widely used in dedicated imaging suites, and the smaller mobile units can be moved by hand to wherever a procedure requiring imaging takes place. These systems are commonly known as C-arms, fluoroscopes, image intensifiers (IIs; technically the name of the receptor rather than the system itself), or by other such names. However, the term 'C-arm' will be used in this book.

A C-arm system features an imaging receptor head that receives the signal transmitted through the region of the patient placed within the beam from the X-ray tube. These are mounted on the opposite ends of a C-shaped support. The receptor head has two functions: to amplify the transmitted X-ray signal so as to allow lower radiation exposure, and to convert the signal to a form that can be immediately displayed and stored. This is often performed by an image intensifier (II) system, although flat panel detector (FPD) heads are now becoming more widely available. Both systems will be covered here.

A standard mobile C-arm system will also include a set of monitors to display images, controls for setting the exposure ranges and storing/recalling images, and warning systems that indicate the emission of radiation. All systems allow the production of both still X-ray images (albeit at reduced dose and image quality) and live fluoroscopic imaging (also known as 'screening' or 'fluoro').

2.1 X-ray tube and generator

Modern mobile C-arm systems do not require a specialized power supply, and so can be run from ordinary wall sockets. Typically, these systems have a multi-phase generator, mounted either on the base unit or C-arm unit (where it can be used to counterbalance the C-arm extension), which supplies consistent power to the X-ray tube. The specifications vary with the model of C-arm, but they may feature high-frequency pulsed exposure settings (e.g. for vascular angiography runs) and lower current continuous output for general fluoroscopy. The generator also supplies high-voltage current to the II head, which requires a very stable and constant power supply to maintain image quality.

The X-ray tube for the C-arm system also varies with regard to system specifications. To allow the system to be mobile (and for the C-arm to be moved by hand), it needs to be as light and small as possible. Systems that can be used to perform vascular imaging will feature rotating anodes (as the tube output is increased for angiography runs, which affects the heat generated at the anode), and may also feature separate focal spots for low- and high-dose imaging. The anode angle will be matched to the focus–film distance (FFD) of the C-arm to avoid any inconsistencies in the beam due to the anode heel effect, while still allowing as steep an angle as possible. This reduces the effective focal spot size, allowing for sharper images to be generated.

Within the beam path, there is a series of lead collimators (often an Iris ring and two linear blades) that allows for the shaping and control of the X-ray beam. This gives the user the ability to collimate areas that would negatively affect the exposure (such as areas of high contrast to the region of interest), to reduce the amount of scattered radiation that would blur the image detail and increase the dose to the patient and staff, and to avoid irradiating sensitive structures that do not need to be demonstrated. However, it is important to be aware of the risks of collimating structures that need to be demonstrated, especially if the region or C-arm has been moved between exposures.

Adjacent to the collimators is the ionization chamber for the dose area product (DAP) meter that is used to measure the radiation output and patient dose. A laser alignment unit may also be mounted around or to the tube, for use as a centring guide.

All of this (with the exception of the beam window) is mounted in a lead-lined casing, which should also protect the X-ray tube from damage and liquids. It also counterbalances the receptor head, to make the C-arm easier to rotate and lessen the strain on the movements and locks.

2.2 Movements and locks

During surgical procedures, the patient is positioned for surgical access rather than ease of imaging. To allow good images to be obtained, mobile C-arm systems are designed to be as versatile as possible with regard to positioning. The movements and adjustments built into the system allow the C-arm to be orientated in almost any direction, and so give a wide range

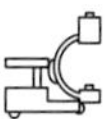

of flexibility in centring (Figure 2.1). While there are limits to what can be achieved, if the patient and equipment are positioned correctly, then, in the majority of cases a good image can be produced. Remember, while it is ideal to get the perfect image straightaway, there is rarely any harm in adjusting the C-arm to improve the image.

The base unit is mounted on wheels that allow free movement or steering. The steering controls fix the unit's movement in one direction, and so keep the centring along a desired path. This can be used, for example, by

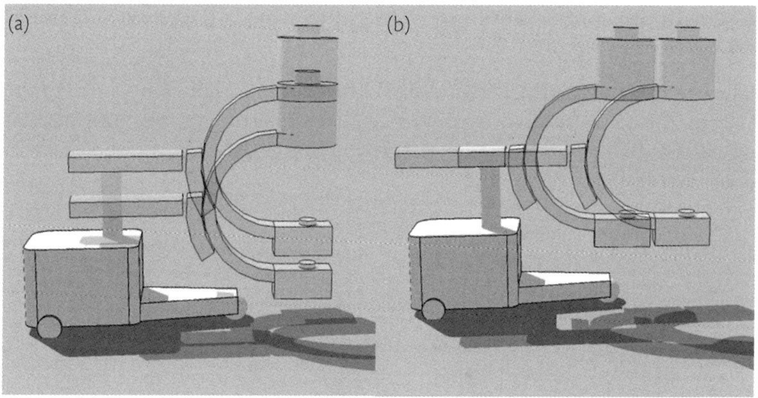

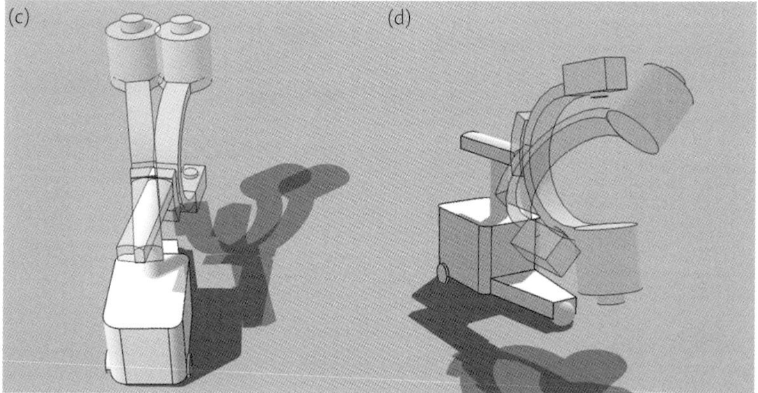

Figure 2.1 C-arm movements. (a) Vertical movement of the C-arm. (b) Back/forth movement of the C-arm. (c) Left/right angulation. (d) Rotation to over/under-couch tube.

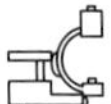

changing the direction of movement to parallel with the patient's femur so as to image from the hip down to the knee while keeping the central beam in the midline of the femur. It also features wheel brakes to prevent unwanted or unintended movement of the C-arm (Figure 2.2).

The centre column can be moved up and down to adjust the height of the C-arm, and can be used to change the object–film distance (OFD). The FFD from the anode to the receptor is normally fixed in mobile units. It can be used for raising the X-ray tube over objects that would impede centring. When changing the height of the C-arm, carefully ensure that the receptor and the tube do not strike any equipment or area of the patient, especially any surgical hardware in use when moving the receptor closer to the patient!

The centre column also allows a small degree of left–right adjustment of the C-arm. This can be used for minor centring adjustments, but one must be aware that this will change the orientation of the receptor as it moves in an arc rather than a straight line.

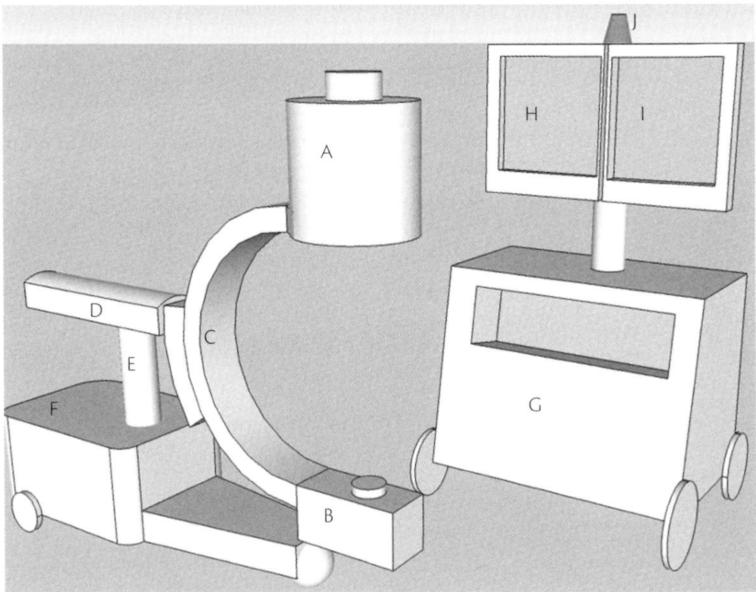

Figure 2.2 C-arm. (a) Intensifier head (II). (b) X-ray tube. (c) C-arm mount. (d) Column extension. (e) Centre column. (f) Control panel on base unit. (g) Monitor station. (h) and (i) Monitors (review and live image). (j) Exposure warning light.

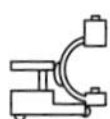

The C-arm is mounted on a sliding extension at the top of the centre column, which gives movement to and from the control panel. It is good practice to slide the extension out halfway before the C-arm is moved into position, as this allows for adjustment in the positioning by moving the sliding extension rather than the entire unit.

Along the sliding extension, there is an axle joint that allows the C-arm assembly to rotate sideways. This movement rotates in both directions, although it is important to be aware of the cables connecting the C-arm to the base unit when turning to prevent damage. This movement allows the C-arm to be orientated in the over-couch position or to give oblique views.

Finally, there is a sliding movement along the curve of the C-arm. This allows the receptor head to be angled up to 90° from vertical towards the base unit (for horizontal beam views), and a varying amount in the opposite direction. Some models allow full rotation to the horizontal beam in both directions, while others are more limited. However, all will allow rotation to the horizontal beam in at least one direction.

All these movements feature locks to prevent accidental movement, and these should be checked regularly. Similarly, the movements should not take an excessive amount of effort when unlocked. Any resistance when moving the C-arm may indicate that the machine is striking or caught on other equipment.

When moving the C-arm to recentre the image, it is possible to become disoriented with the relation between the C-arm movements and the alignment of the patient. This can be due to the lack of visible landmarks on the patient, the contralateral approach of the C-arm, and so on. One technique to overcome this is to attempt to see the relation of the patient to the room, and adjust the C-arm in this aspect rather than from the image. For example, if the lateral aspect of the patients' ankle is facing the scrub room doors, moving the C-arm slightly towards the scrub room doors will recentre the image more laterally on the limb.

2.3 **Image orientation**

All C-arms have mechanisms by which the resulting image can be correctly orientated on the display monitor. This may involve rotating the image (or, in earlier machines, physically turning the receptor), or marking out the direction towards the patient's head. This allows both the surgeons and the radiographer to make their adjustments knowing which directions on the image relate to directions in regard to the patient.

Most systems also feature one or more image reversal settings (along x-axis and y-axis). These can be useful if the C-arm is used in the tube-over-couch position, which will reverse the image on the monitors.

It is sometimes useful to change the orientation of images during the procedure (e.g. if the C-arm approach changes). These adjustments can be made along with centring and collimation adjustments as the procedure progresses.

3

Image receptors

The receptor head is the system that converts the X-ray beam into a visible image and allows it to be displayed. Originally, a phosphor screen was used (along with reduced lighting in the theatre); however, modern systems use either an image intensifier (II) or a flat panel detector (FPD). Both allow real-time fluoroscopy, as well as last-image hold, image storage and retrieval, and other features to assist in procedures or reduce radiation dose. Due to the method by which the old phosphor screen systems worked, the greyscale images were inverted when compared with X-rays (denser items appear darker rather than brighter).

3.1 Image intensifiers

In an II head, the incident X-ray beam is converted into several different forms during the process of amplification. The beam first passes through the input window of the II and strikes the input phosphor, which receives the incident beam that has been transmitted through the patient and converts it to a corresponding pattern of light. This phosphor must absorb and convert as much of the incident beam as possible to improve the efficiency of the system. To do this, the phosphor needs to be as thick as allowable (as greater thickness increases the chances of X-ray photons being converted to light), and it must be made from as dense a material as possible (as denser materials will absorb and convert more beam energy). It should also be sensitive to the energy ranges produced by the X-ray tube (around 50–120 kV). It is typically made of sodium-activated caesium iodide in a series of needle-shaped crystals. These crystals act as 'light pipes', allowing a thicker layer of phosphor to be used while avoiding defocusing as the light is internally reflected along the length of the crystal without diverging. To improve the transmission of the light signal, these crystals are applied directly to the next stage of the II process, the photocathode (Figure 3.1).

The photocathode is a charged plate of antimony–caesium compound that releases electrons when struck by light emitted from the input phosphor.

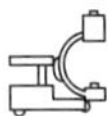

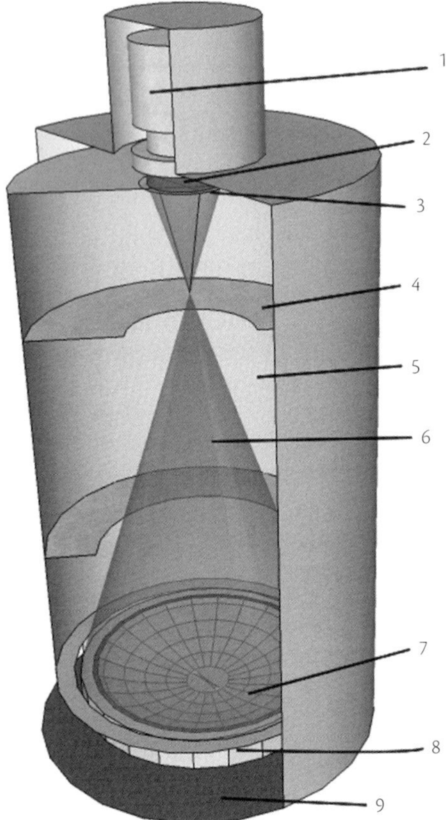

Figure 3.1 Intensifier head cut-away. (1) Camera. (2) Output phosphor. (3) Aluminium window. (4) Focusing magnets. (5) Inner casing/vacuum bottle. (6) Electron beam path. (7) Photocathode. (8) Input phosphor. (9) Incident beam window.

This material is used as it is sensitive to the light spectra released from the input phosphor. The combination of phosphor–photocathode allows a single incident X-ray photon to release around 200 electrons.

The incident X-ray beam has now been converted to an amplified pattern of electrons corresponding to the original incidental beam, which, using a series of charged 'electron lenses', is then accelerated and focused along a cathode ray tube within a vacuum that occupies the bulk of the II head.

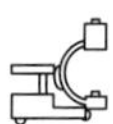

The electron beam is focused onto an output phosphor layer, a small disc that converts the cathode ray beam into visible light, which is then read by the camera system. Similar to the input phosphor, it is constructed as a set of thin, needle-shaped crystals. The phosphor chemistry used is different from that of the input phosphor, as it must be sensitive to different radiations (a cathode beam at around 25 kV, as opposed to X-ray photons at 50–120 kV). It is mounted behind a thin aluminium window at the end of the II head, which allows the cathode ray beam to pass through but reflects emitted light back towards the camera, preventing it from entering the vacuum bottle where it could cause image artefacts.

The output phosphor is connected to a recording system by means of an optical coupler. This is a set of lenses that focus the image onto the recording medium. Older C-arm systems would often feature a set of mirrors that would allow multiple image recording systems to receive the signal, depending on the type of imaging being performed (e.g. a film–screen system for high-resolution runs and a video tube for low-dose fluoroscopy). With advancements in digital imaging systems, a single digital receptor is typically used for both fluoroscopy and spot images.

In some systems, a light-controlling iris is mounted on the path of the light signal. This can close and open to allow less or more light to pass through, respectively. It may seem counterintuitive to reduce the amount of light striking the camera when the entire purpose of the II head is to amplify the X-ray signal as far as possible (and so reduce patient dose). However, when very high-quality images are required (e.g. cardiac angiography runs), the X-ray tube output must be increased to improve the signal-to-noise ratio (SNR). The amplification from the II head is fixed (assuming magnification settings remain the same). This means that the II head will put out very clear, well-defined images with little noise, but images that are so bright as to totally overwhelm the camera. Closing the iris therefore allows the camera to receive enough light to generate a good image without saturation that would cause overexposure and loss of detail (Van Lysel 2000). Digital matrix sensors tend to have a more linear sensitivity that can handle a wider range of exposure without signal loss, and so these systems may not feature a light-controlling iris. See the 'Exposures and image quality' section for more detail.

The camera itself can be used to gauge the exposure required from the X-ray tube by sensing the amount of light entering it and comparing that with a reference exposure, increasing the tube output if more exposure is required and decreasing it if less. Alternatively, a photosensor can be attached to the optical coupling to monitor light output from the output phosphor to perform the same task (Geise 2001). More modern systems can analyse the image itself and compensate for very dark or bright areas and so adjust the exposure to better demonstrate the useful mid-range of the image. The recording mechanism used should feature the highest spatial resolution achievable, and also as little delay in the imaging chain (known as 'lag') as possible, since this will cause blurring of moving structures from the residual signal. This will allow good temporal and spatial resolutions for the entire system.

The input phosphor and photocathode form a convex dome behind the input window on the front of the II. This maintains a constant distance between the photocathode and the (flat) output phosphor across its diameter, so as to keep a single point of focus for the converging beam. It also acts as a strong barrier against the pressure differences between the II head (which is a vacuum so as to allow the cathode beam to flow unimpeded) and the surrounding environment. This setup can cause drop-off of signals around the edges (and so a darkening of the image), known as 'vignetting'. It can also distort the images generated by the II, and so the imaging chain is often designed to compensate for such distortions. The equipment should be periodically checked for image distortion and vignetting via QA tests.

Within the outer casing is a layer of lead shielding that absorbs scattered radiation within the head, and prevents external scatter or radiation sources from affecting the image. Underneath this is a layer of mu-metal that blocks external magnetic interference. The focusing electrodes of the II magnetically focus the electron beam onto the output phosphor, so external fields can cause distortions on the image. Within this is the vacuum bottle that allows the cathode beam to flow across the II unimpeded.

These are all housed in a shielded metal casing that protects the inner workings of the intensifier, featuring attachments for an X-ray grid in front of the input window, laser alignment units, and so on, and also for attaching the II head onto the C-arm assembly. The outer casing should be easy to clean, and must be strong enough to protect the workings of the II head from everyday wear and tear (Schueler 2000).

3.2 Intensification

The signal amplification in an II system happens in two stages. The first occurs at the phosphors and photocathode. A single X-ray photon striking the input phosphor may produce hundreds of emitted electrons from the photocathode. Similarly, a single accelerated electron striking the output phosphor may cause thousands of light photons to be emitted. For example, one incident X-ray photon can be converted into 200 photoelectrons, which then

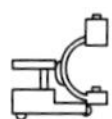

release up to 2000 light photons each at the output phosphor, amplifying the signal 400,000 times. In actual practice, however, due to inefficiencies in the conversion chain, the actual amplification is closer to 100 times the input. This is known as 'flux'.

The second method of amplification is the condensing of the cathode beam down from a large input (e.g. 22 cm diameter or 380 cm^2 area) to a much smaller output (e.g. 2 cm diameter or 3.14 cm^2 area), so that the same signal is focused into a more concentrated beam. This process is called 'minification'. The amplification from minification is calculated by the input field size (380) divided by the output field size (3), and so the signal is amplified approximately 120 times. The total amount of signal intensification is therefore flux (100) × minification (120) = 12,000. Put another way, the video camera can receive the same image with the intensifier using 1/12000th of the exposure that would be needed if just a phosphor plate was used to convert the beam to light (Wang and Blackburn 2000).

Modern C-arm systems feature electronic magnification modes. In II systems, this works by narrowing the X-ray beam to a smaller diameter using the iris collimator, then refocusing the II head to the region of the input phosphor that is exposed so that all the output phosphor is still covered. This process increases the spatial resolution of the images acquired, allowing for finer details to be visualized (albeit over a smaller area). However, as the exposed area of the input phosphor shrinks, so does the ratio between the input and output phosphor sizes, and so the minification factor decreases. This means that the X-ray tube output has to increase to maintain the same output from the II head to the camera, increasing the entrance skin dose (ESD). The general rule is that the dose increases (or decreases) by the square of the ratio of the input beam sizes. Therefore, going from a 20-cm-diameter field to a 10-cm-diameter field would increase the entrance skin dose four times: (20/10)2 = 4 (Mahesh 2001). As such, it is advisable to use electronic magnification sparingly.

3.3 Flat-panel detectors

A relatively recent development is the wider use of FPDs as opposed to II heads for C-arm systems. Though predominantly used in fixed-location systems (e.g. vascular labs), mobile C-arm systems are becoming available with FPD image receptors. These systems operate by having a matrix of individual detector elements (DELs) that receive energy from the incident beam either directly in X-ray form, or after conversion to light via a scintillation phosphor of needle-shaped, thallium-activated, caesium–iodide crystals. These two systems are known as 'direct' and 'indirect', respectively. Each

DEL acts as a semiconductor that allows current to flow into a capacitor in proportion to the incidental exposure. A control system then reads the charges of each DEL row by row, the outputted charge is amplified, and the values across the detector are translated into an image. Therefore, each DEL acts as a single pixel within the outputted image.

Due to the much simpler conversion chain when compared with IIs, there is much less opportunity for distortion and noise to develop. For example, the uniformity of the system across the incidental beam (unlike the curved input phosphor in an II) prevents vignetting and defocusing, and the lack of cathode ray projection helps avoid pincushion or S distortions from voltage fluctuations or external magnetic fields. The FPD system also directly outputs a digital signal without the need to convert via a charged coupled device (CCD) camera. Typically, the CCD camera in an II has a much narrower dynamic range than the intensifier itself, and so an aperture within the optical coupling is used to keep the output phosphor's signal within the range of the CCD camera. However, an FPD can receive a much wider range and display it directly, so that images that would have areas of saturation on an II system may still have good levels of detail. The fewer stages of conversion and lack of projection within the detector also mean that an FPD receptor can be much smaller and lighter than an II head.

As the size of the DELs is fixed, so too is the maximum spatial resolution of an FPD system. Magnification modes are available on FPD systems, but the spatial resolution does not increase with each mag step as in an II system. Instead, the beam is collimated into the new field size, and the exposed area on the detector is enlarged to fill the entire display screen so that each DEL represents a larger region of the screen. As there is no loss of minification gain in mag modes for an FPD system, there is also no direct need to increase the tube output when using these modes. However, as the inherent noise in the detector does become more visible when the images are enlarged, many manufacturers still increase the tube output for mag modes to improve the SNR and reduce noise. The increase in exposure is typically less than that used in an II system (Nickoloff 2011) (Figure 3.2).

Depending on the number of DELs and the required frame rate, the control systems for an FPD must be able to receive data at very high rates (around 240Mb/s is not uncommon). Some systems (when not using magnification modes) use a process called 'binning', where a number of DELs in a square are averaged out and so sent as a single pixel. This can hugely reduce the volume of data the system needs to process, at the cost of reducing spatial resolution.

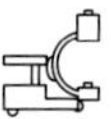

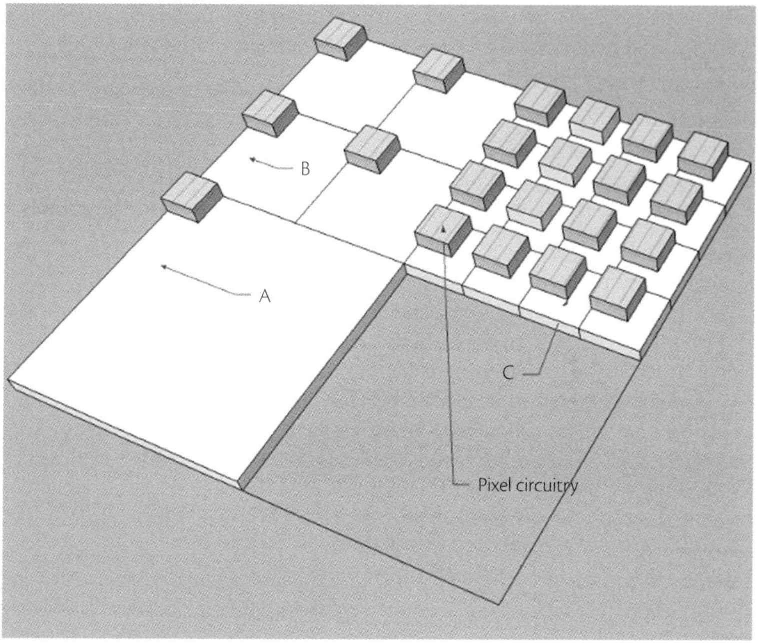

Figure 3.2 Flat-panel sensor example with three different detector element (DEL) sizes. Note how the pixel circuitry is the same size but takes up a greater ratio of the DEL in the smaller DEL sizes (C) than the larger ones. As such, (C) will have better spatial resolution than (B) or (A), while (A) will have much greater radiation sensitivity than (B) or (C).

As DEL size relates to the spatial resolution of an FPD system, it would seem a good idea to make them as small as possible for better image detail. However, there are difficulties inherent with producing smaller DELs, the first being that smaller DELs typically have less efficiency in converting incident beam to output signal. Not all the area of a DEL is used to receive incident beams, as each has connectors and control circuitry that occupies a certain area of the DEL itself. This area is known as the 'dead area', and the ratio of DEL size to actual beam detecting area of the DEL is known as the 'fill factor', with the ideal being 1, but more typically being around 0.6–0.8. As the area of the DEL is reduced, the dead area typically remains the same size (these circuits are normally already as small as can be reliably manufactured), taking up proportionally more area of the DEL, reducing the fill factor and hence the sensitivity. Smaller DELs are also harder (and

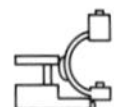

more expensive) to manufacture, as the required tolerances in production get finer, and hence smaller errors have larger effects on the image quality.

Although FPDs are far less sensitive to magnetic fields and voltage fluctuations than II heads, they are still sensitive to temperature and physical damage. Damaged or defective DELs can affect image quality, and although most systems have interpolation software to counter these effects, once enough DELs become defective, the image quality will degrade noticeably.

Some studies have found that ESD compared between cardiac II and FPD systems do not vary significantly (Chida et al. 2009). However, the use of low-dose acquisition modes that feature on many newer FPD systems can apparently reduce patient dose when compared with older II-based interventional units, while maintaining a comparable image quality. Several studies have compared systems for dose and image quality in either clinical settings or using anatomical phantoms, and have achieved lower dose rates using the newer FPD systems with dose-reduction settings. Exactly how much of these savings are due to the FPD system itself as opposed to the replacement of old equipment with more modern systems is unclear. More modern systems (both FPD and II) may also have more advanced dose-optimization software and a greater range of reduced-exposure settings that can reduce the radiation dose when compared with older equipment. Studies comparing the relationship between dose and image quality between FPD and II systems have so far concluded that radiation dose does not vary significantly between the systems at comparable image quality levels. As of today, it is probably simplest to say that FPD systems may have a potential advantage in reducing radiation dose to patients and theatre staff (especially in magnification modes), although it is by no means guaranteed (Bogaert et al. 2008; Hatakeyama et al. 2007; Suzuki et al. 2005; Tsapaki et al. 2004).

References

Bogaert, E., Bacher, K., Lapere, R., and Thierens, H. 'Does Digital Flat Detector Technology Tip the Scale Towards Better Image Quality or Reduced Patient Dose in Interventional Cardiology?', *European Journal of Radiology*, 72/2 (2008), 348–53. doi:10.1016/j.ejrad.2008.07.028.

Chida, K., Inaba, Y., Saito, H., Ishibashi, T., Takahashi, S., Kohzuki, M., and Zuguchi, M. Radiation Dose of Interventional Radiology System Using a Flat-Panel Detector. *American Journal of Roentgenology*, 193/6 (2009), 1680–85.

Geise, R. A. 'The AAPM/RSNA Physics Tutorial for Residents—Fluoroscopy: Recording of Fluoroscopic Images and Automatic Exposure Control', *Radiographics*, 21/1 (2001), 227–36.

Hatakeyama, Y., Kakeda, S., Ohnari, N., Moriya, J., Oda, N., Nishino, K., Miyamoto, W., and Korogi, Y. 'Reduction of Radiation Dose for Cerebral Angiography Using

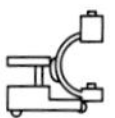

Flat Panel Detector of Direct Conversion Type: A Vascular Phantom Study', *American Journal of Neuroradiology*, 26/8 (2007), 645–50.

Mahesh, M. 'The AAPM/RSNA Physics Tutorial for Residents—Fluoroscopy: Patient Radiation Exposure Issues', *Radiographics*, 21/4 (2001), 1033–45.

Nickoloff, E. 'AAPM/RSNA Physics Tutorial for Residents: Physics of Flat-Panel Fluoroscopy Systems', *Radiographics*, 31/2 (2011), 591–602.

Schueler, B. A. 'The AAPM/RSNA Physics Tutorial for Residents—General Overview of Fluoroscopic Imaging', *Radiographics*, 20/4 (2000), 1115–26.

Suzuki, S., Furui, S., Kobayashi, I., Yamauchi, T., Kohtake, H., Takeshita, K., Takada, K., and Yamagishi, M. 'Radiation Dose to Patients and Radiologists During Transcatheter Arterial Embolization: Comparison of a Digital Flat-Panel System and Conventional Unit', *American Journal of Radiology*, 185/4 (2005), 855–59.

Tsapaki, V., Kottou, S., Kollaros, N., Dafnomili, P., Koutelou, M., Vano, E., and Neofotistou, V. 'Comparison of a Conventional and a Flat-Panel Digital System in Interventional Cardiology Procedures', *The British Journal of Radiology*, 77/919 (2004), 562–67.

Van Lysel, M. 'The AAPM/RSNA Physics Tutorial for Residents—Fluoroscopy: Optical Coupling and the Video System', *Radiographics*, 20/6 (2000), 1769–86.

Wang, J. and Blackburn, T. 'The AAPM/RSNA Physics Tutorial for Residents—X-ray Image Intensifiers for Fluoroscopy', *Radiographics*, 20/5 (2000), 1471–77.

4

Exposures and image quality

In C-arm systems, the X-ray beam output is determined by both the signal returned from the automatic exposure device (AED) in the receptor and the exposure table set up for the exam type. The exposure table acts as a reference for the range of exposures that will give a good image for the selected exam, while the AED adjusts the level along the table that is used. Specific exposure tables may be set up for orthopaedics, spinal procedures, paediatrics, procedures involving iodinated contrast, and so on. The settings for the exposure (as well as aspects of the image receptor and display) will affect the qualities or resolutions of the resulting image. The outputted image display may also be adjusted for brightness and contrast by the windowing settings built into the C-arm system. However, for this section, the focus will be on image generation rather than display.

The three resolutions are *spatial* (the minimum size of items that can be visualized), *contrast* (how much structures need to vary in their density to appear separate on the image), and *temporal* (the timescale an image covers, and so how much movement blur can be accepted). All these resolutions are related to the radiation exposure and the dose to the patient and theatre staff. As such, under the principles of 'as low as reasonably practicable' (ALARP), it is important for the radiographer to understand resolutions to be able to minimize dose to the patient and staff.

4.1 Spatial resolution

'Spatial resolution' refers to how small a structure can be clearly demonstrated by the imaging system. The greater the resolution of a system, the finer the details that can be seen on images produced by it. Imagine placing a grid of squares over a photograph, and averaging the contents of each square down to a single colour. Obviously, the smaller (and more numerous) the squares, the more this image will resemble the original photo, whereas fewer larger squares will result in a less detailed image. The spatial resolution is generally inherent in the systems used in the whole imaging chain (the receptor head and camera if applicable, whether any compression algorithm is employed,

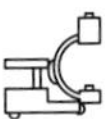

and the output monitors). In image intensifier (II) systems, the spatial resolution is typically determined by the camera system attached to the output phosphor and the magnification setting (in magnification modes, the camera resolution remains the same but it covers a smaller area, thus increasing the effective resolution). In flat-panel detector (FPD) systems, the spatial resolution is fixed due to the size of the detector elements (DELs), but it can be reduced by binning). Distortion effects and poorly maintained display systems can also affect the spatial resolution and should be checked for regularly via QA testing. Generally, mobile C-arm systems are not used to visualize very fine detail, and so can have a lower spatial resolution than plain film or vascular lab systems.

What is also important regarding spatial resolution is the level of noise in the image (background static–like effects on the image). Noise is an inherent factor in all receptors that degrades image quality, being an entirely random pattern that appears on images. The relationship between background noise and image is known as the 'signal-to-noise ratio' (SNR). Higher signal strength (i.e. more exposure transmitted through the patient) dilutes the effect of noise, increasing the image quality at the expense of a higher radiation dose. Where large structures are being viewed and very fine detail is not a priority, a lower SNR can be acceptable as the noise will not affect the outcome from the image. However, where image quality is a priority (such as when visualizing small blood vessels in angiography), a much higher SNR (and therefore dose) is required to prevent noise artefacts from degrading important structural details.

Spatial resolution is measured in visible line pairs per millimetre (lp/mm). This is measured by placing a phantom containing high contrast bands of attenuating material in a range of widths, and then judging the width at which the individual bands are no longer clearly demonstrated on the resulting image. As the entire imaging chain (receptor through to output monitors) can affect the clarity of spatial resolution, any clear deterioration picked up in Quality Assurance will need to be checked further to isolate the elements or combination of elements that are degrading the image quality.

4.2 Contrast resolution

Within the sensitivity ranges of whichever receptor system is used, the balance between kVp and mA is reciprocal. This means the same exposure at the receptor can be obtained by either a smaller number of high-energy photons that can penetrate structures (high kVp, low mAs), or with a larger number of low-energy photons to achieve enough penetration through structures

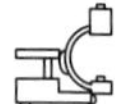

(low kVp, high mAs). All things being equal, it would be preferable to always use higher-kVp techniques, as this gives a lower dose to the patient while still generating an image. However, the use of higher kVp also reduces image contrast, as structures of differing densities will appear the same on the final image. There is therefore a trade-off between dose and contrast, where structures with large differences in density (e.g. compact bone and soft tissue) can be demonstrated well using high kVp, whereas structures with less difference (such as regions of soft tissue) will require lower kVp to improve the contrast between structures (Mahesh 2001) (Figure 4.1).

Because of this, modern C-arm systems have exposure tables that allow different exposure settings, depending on the type of imaging being performed. For example, where good soft-tissue contrast is not as important, or where dose must be minimized (e.g. appendicular orthopaedics and paediatrics, respectively), a higher kVp with less mA will be used than where a good contrast range is more important. Other systems may have specific settings for iodine contrast studies where the kVp is set at the level that gives best contrast while the mA varies to produce enough exposure to form an image. The AED system reads the level of signal obtained by the receptor and adjusts the exposure up or down the exposure curve as necessary. In

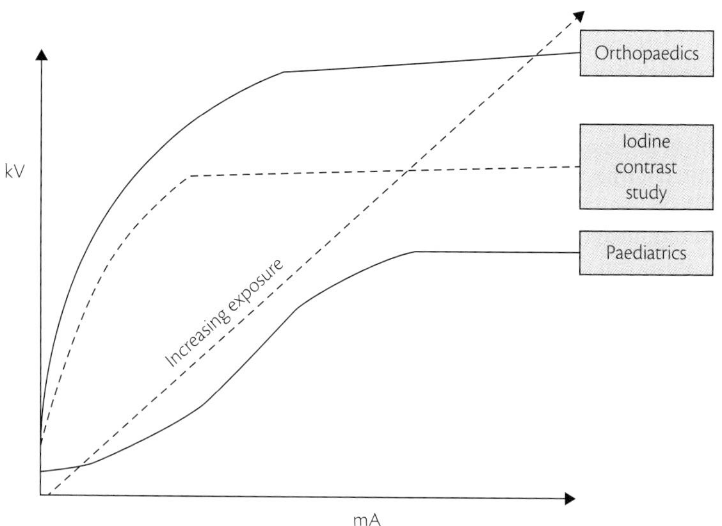

Figure 4.1 Example of exposure curves. Note the iodine curve peaks at kV that best demonstrate the iodine contrast.

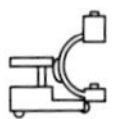

older II systems, the signal would be read using a light sensor built into the optical coupling, measuring the light generated by the output phosphor (Reilly and Sutton 2001). More modern systems, however, perform an analysis of the digital image itself, taking into account and compensating for the extremes of the image range, such as beam-occluding artefacts.

4.3 **Temporal resolution**

One of the main advantages of the C-arm system is that it allows for the real-time viewing of movement by taking a rapid succession of low-dose images. 'Temporal resolution' can be defined as how long it takes to obtain a single image, similar to the shutter speed on a camera. A high temporal resolution will acquire each image over a very short period, and so can show an object moving clearly, whereas a lower resolution will make the movement appear blurred as there is more movement of the structure while the image is being obtained. Once again though, higher temporal resolution comes at the expense of a higher dose to the patient. For the receptor to achieve sufficient signal to produce an image, a set amount of radiation must strike it. For example, assuming that a resolution of 10 images (or frames) per second is needed, the tube will need to emit enough radiation to generate an image every 1/10th of a second. (Note: This is why C-arm systems typically state exposure factors in mA rather than mAs as with plain film systems. The exposure time continues as long as the expose button is pressed.) In II head systems, the maximum temporal resolution is normally defined by the afterglow time of the output phosphor (how long the phosphor crystals continue to produce light after the electron beam has stopped) and the lag in the camera/video-tube system. In FPD systems, it is dependent on the input phosphor afterglow (if an indirect system is used) and the data transfer rate of the receptor.

Where movements of structures do not need to be demonstrated, savings can be made in dose by lowering the temporal resolution and averaging out images over time. C-arm systems typically have reduced dose settings, where the pulse rate of the tube is dropped and the generated image is created by averaging lower exposure images. These settings can greatly reduce exposure, but any movement of the structures being imaged will produce blurring on the final image (as movement occurs between frames that are then combined). Even minor vibrations of the C-arm can cause noticeable degradation of the image when using the lowest pulse setting. As such, it is normally a good idea to allow the machine a few seconds to settle after moving before attempting images in low-dose pulsed exposure modes (Figure 4.2).

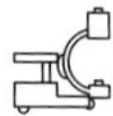

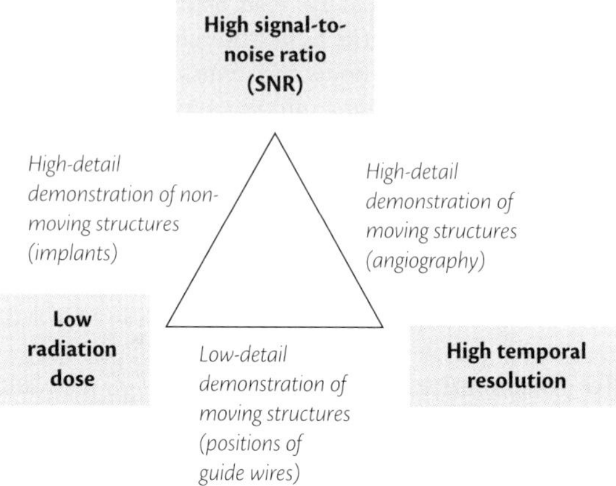

Figure 4.2 Relationship between different factors affecting image quality and radiation dose. Only two factors can be applicable at a time, so a decision must be made depending on the requirements of the structures being imaged at the time.

In simple terms, generating an image is a trade-off between the desire for high SNR, high temporal resolution, and low dose (all within the required contrast range). At best, only two of these factors can be achieved, and it is the duty of the radiographer to prioritize the most important factors at the time. Some examples are:

- *Demonstrating the position of an orthopaedic implant.* No movement, so no need for high temporal resolution.
- *Inserting a catheter over a guidewire up the ureter into the kidney before contrast is injected.* Fine detail not needed, so no need for high SNR.
- *Visualizing branches of the coronary artery under contrast injection.* Involves small, rapidly moving structures that must be clearly demonstrated, so higher exposure and (hence) higher dose will be required.

4.4 Under- and overexposure

All C-arm systems feature AEDs that monitor the output from the receptor and adjust the X-ray output accordingly. However, these systems are not infallible and may adjust the exposure incorrectly if much of the image is taken up by either beam-blocking artefacts or empty space. These may cause the system to compensate by increasing or decreasing the exposure, respectively,

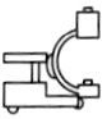

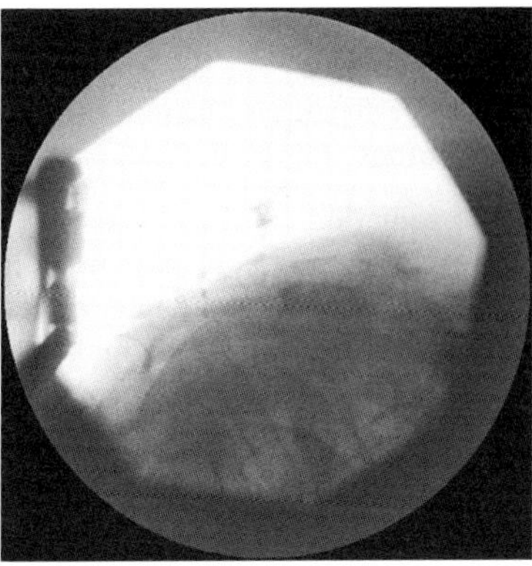

Figure 4.3 Poor exposure due to excessive contrast between dense region and air. Good collimation would produce a more usable image.
Reproduced courtesy of Radiology Department, Leeds Teaching Hospitals NHS Trust, UK.

to try and average out the exposure across the image, causing over- or under-exposure of the region of interest (Figure 4.3).

The exposure can be corrected and these issues avoided by removing all beam-blocking artefacts from the beam path (by either physically removing them or adjusting the C-arm position to move them out of the beam path), judiciously using collimators to shape the beam around the region of interest, and avoiding areas of high contrast in the image. If necessary, manual exposure settings can also be used. However, all three techniques have their limits. For example, some beam-blocking artefacts may not be removable from the region of interest (such as surgical hardware or supports). Collimators may clip off regions that need to be demonstrated, especially if there is any movement between images. Manual exposures may increase the patients' dose by necessitating several exposures with adjustments before a good image is produced, and will not automatically reduce the exposure if any obstructions are removed (although the imaging system will compensate to produce a good image, the exposure will be higher than necessary; as such, this is not advisable under ALARP principles).

4.5 Scatter

Interactions with tissues can cause X-ray photons to divert from their original path. This is known as 'beam scatter' and can result in an increased radiation dose to the patient (by irradiating tissues outside the primary beam) and to the surgical team (from photons that are deflected out of the patient towards the team members). Scatter can also lead to a loss of detail at the image receptor as the image-forming coherent photons are overlaid with non-coherent scattered photons (Figure 4.4).

The amount of scattered radiation can be affected by the volume of tissue irradiated (larger areas will scatter more photons) and the beam energy (higher exposures will result in greater amounts of scatter). The effects of scatter can best be reduced by irradiating a smaller volume of tissue (via collimation, compression, or angling of the beam so that it does not pass

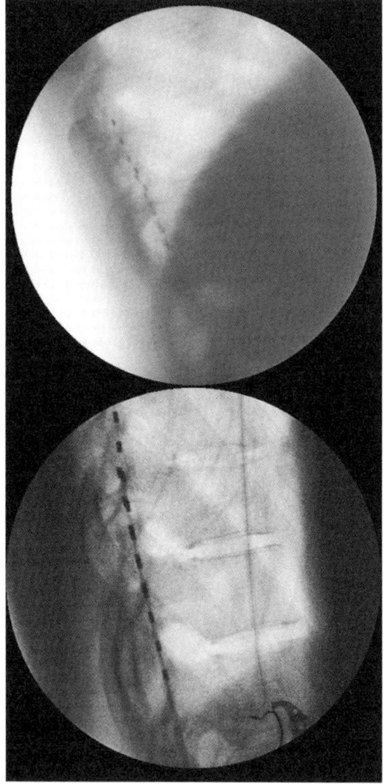

Figure 4.4 Top—Blurred image caused by scattered radiation. **Bottom**—Linear collimation has reduced the volumes of tissue irradiated, and so reduced scatter. Note the clearer definition of vertebrae, visibility of intervertebral spaces.

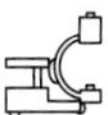

through unnecessary structures). Dose from scatter to the surgical team can be minimized by reducing exposure and maintaining distance from the patient and primary beam while exposures are happening, although this may not always be possible.

Some systems feature an anti-scatter grid attached to the input window of the receptor head, which should be removable and used only when necessary. As with all anti-scatter grids, it will absorb scattered radiation and improve image quality but increase the dose to the patient (Schueler et al. 2006).

4.6 Motion blurring

While all modern C-arm receptors allow real-time live imaging, the images they produce are made up of still images (albeit presented in sequence). If lower frame rates are used to reduce the radiation dose, any movement of the anatomy or C-arm may produce blurred images. While slight movements may blur fine detail and yet be deemed acceptable (such as the trabecular pattern of bone), larger movements may produce images where the anatomy cannot be visualized. As such, this results in a radiation dose to the patient and staff for no reason whatsoever (Figure 4.5).

Under the principles of ALARP, it is a good idea to use as low a frame rate as achievable when using a C-arm system to demonstrate anatomy that is not moving. However, if movement is being demonstrated (e.g. functional views

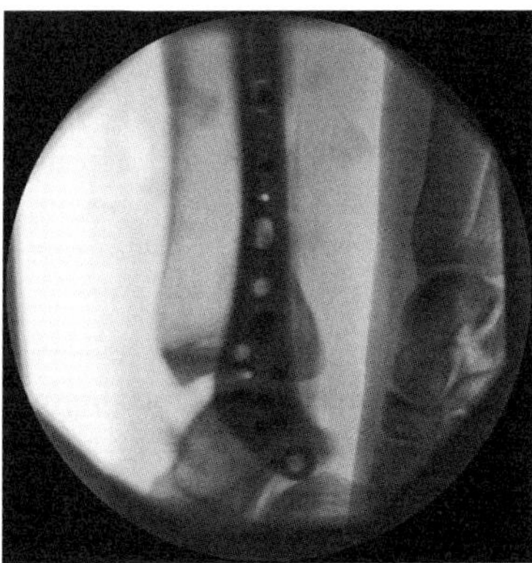

Figure 4.5 Blurring of the ankle plate due to movement of the leg. Note also the sharply defined contralateral ankle included to the right of the image. Having this within the primary beam increases the dose to the patient, and as such is a poor technique.
Reproduced courtesy of Radiology Department, Leeds Teaching Hospitals NHS Trust, UK.

of a joint or contrast flowing along a structure), higher frame rates are required to produce clearer images. Such exposures will generate higher X-ray doses than lower-frame-rate images, and will typically involve longer beam-on times. As such, it is important to stop the exposure as soon as possible to avoid excessive radiation dose to the patient and staff. This is best achieved by good communication with the surgeons. The radiographer may also stop screening once the surgeons look away from the monitors if they are confident that the need for imaging has ceased.

4.7 Distortion

The cathode ray projection system can make II heads prone to image distortion. The most common types are 'pincushion distortion' (where the centre of the image has different magnification than the periphery) and 'S distortion' (where straight lines across the image curve into an 'S' shape around the centre of the image field). Pincushion distortions are caused by de-focusing of the cathode ray projection, whereas S distortions are caused by external magnetic fields. Both can be checked for by imaging a parallel chequerboard grid with the II system, and checking that all the lines on the resulting image are parallel (Figure 4.6).

Over time, the vacuum within the II will degrade, disrupting the path of the cathode beam. As this happens, more electrons will be blocked from striking the output phosphor, and so a higher exposure will be required to create a satisfactory image. X-ray output should be periodically checked using a standardized system of QA, to check for both variations in the tube output and sensitivity of the II head.

Blurring and variations in image size can also occur in II systems. This can be caused by fluctuations in the voltage to the focusing electrodes within the II, causing the cathode ray beam to lose focus on the output phosphor. Distortion can also be a result of problems with the optical coupling and camera, or the monitors mounted on the base unit.

Over time, the edges around the images produced can start to darken. This is known as 'vignetting', and it is most clearly seen on very low exposures (e.g. exposing with nothing in the beam path). Generally, this effect disappears in normal use; however, if it starts affecting image quality, the C-arm should be checked by an engineer.

C-arm systems may, over time, start to lose the capacity to demonstrate fine detail as the images produced become defocused. This loss of spatial resolution can be caused by faults in any part of the imaging chain; as such, once

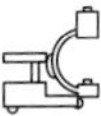

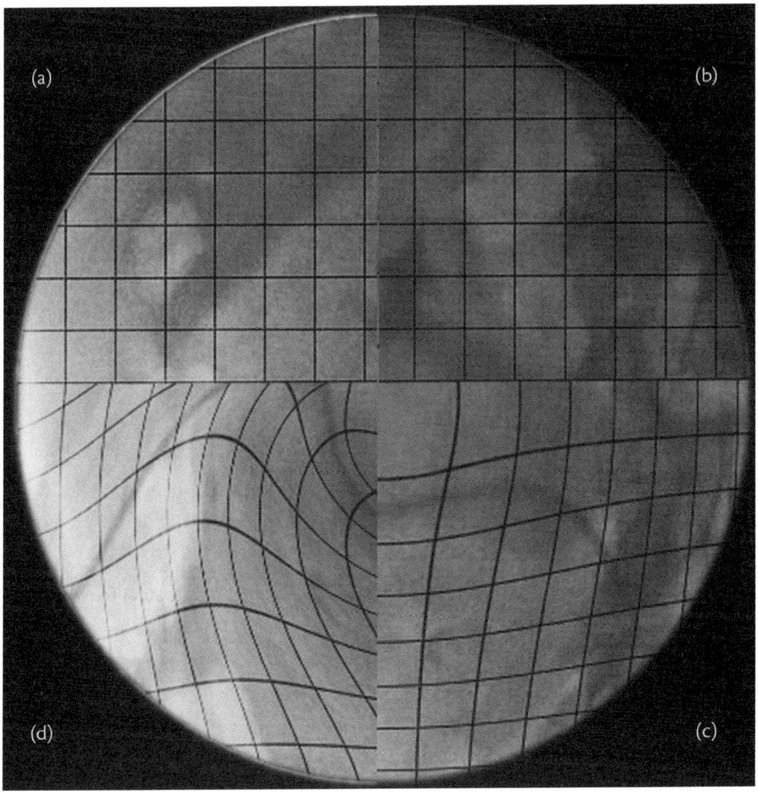

(a) (b) (d) (c)

Figure 4.6 Examples of distortion, clockwise from top left. (a) Normal image (checkerboard pattern added). (b) Vignetting. Note the darkening around edge of image. (c) Pincushion distortion. (d) S distortion.

Reproduced courtesy of Radiology Department, Leeds Teaching Hospitals NHS Trust, UK.

they occur, the equipment should be checked by an engineer. Regular QA checks using a spatial resolution test tool should be performed to check for any loss of focus.

References

Mahesh, M. 'The AAPM/RSNA Physics Tutorial for Residents—Fluoroscopy: Patient Radiation Exposure Issues', *Radiographics*, 21/4 (2001), 1033–45.

Reilly, A. and Sutton, D. 'A Computer Model of an Image Intensifier System Working under Automatic Brightness Control', *The British Journal of Radiology*, 74 (2001), 938–48.

Schueler, B. A., Vrieze, T. J., Bjarnason, H., and Stanson, A. W. 'An Investigation of Operator Exposure in Interventional Radiology', *Radiographics*, 26/5 (2006), 1533–41.

5

Radiation protection

The basics of radiation protection in the theatre for the patient follow principles similar to those used in plain-film imaging. These include ensuring positive identification of the patient, justification of radiation exposure, avoiding irradiation of pregnant patients wherever possible, minimization and optimization of exposures performed (ALARP principle), protection of all staff involved, and recording and monitoring of all exposures performed.

The World Health Organization has set up a protocol for avoiding mistakes in patient and procedure details for surgery. Before the induction of anaesthesia, the patients' identity must be confirmed, consent obtained, and the procedure to be undertaken confirmed. Pregnancy status should also be checked at this stage if applicable to the patient. These details are then repeated to all the theatre staff during the time out (before the start of the procedure). Any uncertainties about radiation protection should be raised as soon as possible to the entire team and be recorded in the procedure notes.

At the end of any case, a record of the radiation exposure should be kept for radiation-monitoring purposes. This normally consists of a dose area product (DAP) reading taken from an ionization chamber mounted in front of the X-ray tube aperture, and the screening (or 'beam-on') time. This allows a record of the patient's exposure to be kept, and issues with radiation exposure (e.g. due to malfunctioning equipment) to be identified (Figure 5.1).

Assuming that exposure factors have been set correctly, there are other factors that will also affect the radiation dose to the patient. The screening time is obviously a major factor, and it should be minimized as far as possible. This can be achieved by accurate positioning and centring before exposing to avoid the need to repeat imaging. All modern systems feature a 'last image hold' (LIH) system, where the last acquired image is displayed on the monitors without any further need for exposure. Saving images regularly also helps avoid the need for re-exposure if the surgeon wishes to compare images. Modern digital C-arm systems have large capacities for storing images, and saved images that do not need to be archived can be discarded at the end of a case.

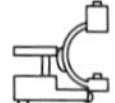

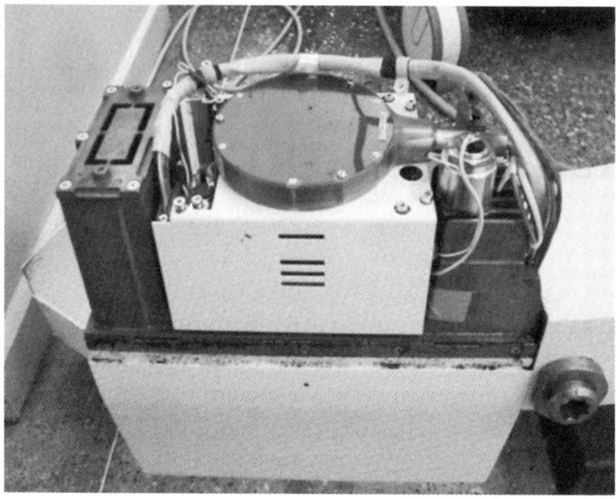

Figure 5.1 DAP meter (circle at top) above white box holding collimators. The X-ray tube is housed in the larger white box below.

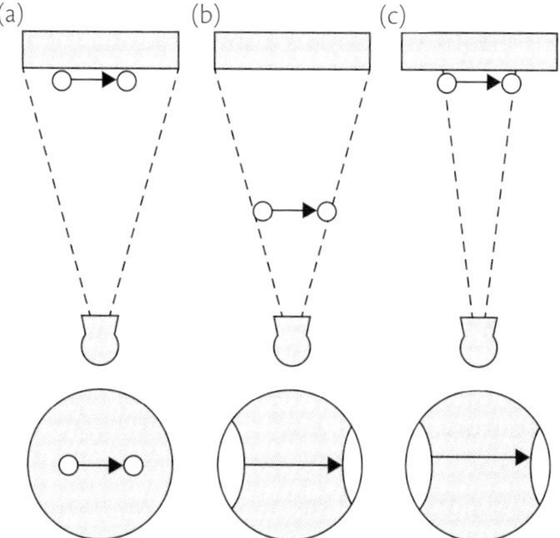

Figure 5.2 Effects of object–film distance (OFD) and magnification modes (mag modes) on movement. (a) Movement of item across receptor head; bottom shows resulting image. (b) Same movement with increased OFD causes object to be magnified and clipped. (c) Same movement on mag mode causes object again to be clipped.

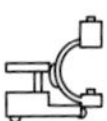

Live screening (also known as 'dynamic imaging'), as opposed to still or flash images, increases patient exposure significantly due to the longer period of exposure. Hence, this should be avoided except where movement has to be demonstrated, and only conducted for as long as is necessary. Good communication with surgeons is the best technique for avoiding unnecessarily long exposures. The radiographer should, however, be aware that surgeons may not state when they are finished with imaging, and as such should stop exposures once surgeons look away from the screen.

Another factor is the distance between the patient and the receptor (object–film distance, or OFD). Ideally, the receptor should be as close as possible to the region of the patient undergoing imaging, as this reduces both geometric magnification and the intensity of the beam passing though the region (as beam intensity reduces with distance in accordance with the inverse-square law). However, it is often necessary to leave a gap between the receptor and the patient to allow the surgeon access to the area. Nevertheless, it is still important to keep the X-ray tube as far from the patient as feasible during exposures (Figure 5.2).

Note: Although it may seem that using the C-arm in an over-couch configuration may allow the receptor to be brought closer to the region of interest (ROI) while allowing the surgeons greater access, this configuration increases back-scatter dose to the surgical team (especially to the eyes and thyroid), and risks damage to the receptor head; therefore, this should be avoided. See the section titled 'Protection for theatre staff' for more information.

The direction of the beam through the patient is an important factor. Oblique views may irradiate a greater volume of tissue than straight anterior–posterior views, thereby increasing the absorbed dose as well as the entrance surface dose (ESD), since the tube will increase output to penetrate the greater volume of tissue. Similarly, lateral views of the abdomen/pelvis should be avoided unless absolutely necessary.

Structures that cause attenuation of the beam will increase tube output, as the AED compensates to maintain acceptable image quality. Some of these structures are, of course, unavoidable (such as the operating table surface), and they are typically made of radio-lucent materials. However, some items used for patient positioning (e.g. sandbags) are not designed to be radio-lucent, and so will cause reduced image quality and an increase in dose. Any such items should either be removed if possible or replaced with a more radio-lucent item. Similarly, anti-scatter grids mounted on the C-arm receptor should be removed when not necessary to maintain image quality. Removal of grids can reduce patient exposure significantly, albeit with an associated increase in scattered radiation striking the receptor (Parry et al. 1999).

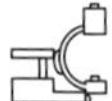

5.1 Collimation and shielding

All modern C-arm systems feature collimators for beam shaping, mounted in the X-ray tube assembly. Typically, these consist of two linear blades and a circular iris. Some systems allow the linear collimators to be moved independently, and so allow very precise beam shaping. Others only allow them to be closed/opened and rotated together. These systems should be used whenever practicable to reduce the volume of tissue irradiated as much as possible, aimed at reducing both the direct dose to the patient as well as the scattered radiation that will increase the dose to other areas of the patient and the surgical team. Where there is frequent movement of either the ROI or C-arm, it is easy to overcollimate by clipping off relevant areas on the resulting image. Radiographers should familiarize themselves with whatever systems they have and use them appropriately (Figure 5.3, Figure 5.4).

Lead shielding can be used on patients for their protection, although it is important to place it in a manner that blocks radiation before it enters the patient—that is, closer to the tube than the receptor. Poorly placed lead protection may reflect X-rays back into the patient rather than offer protection from them.

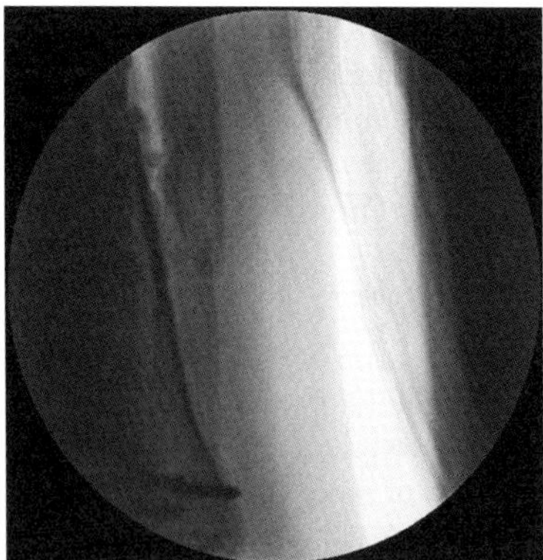

Figure 5.3 Anatomy clipped by linear collimation. Recentring would improve the image.

Reproduced courtesy of Radiology Department, Leeds Teaching Hospitals NHS Trust, UK.

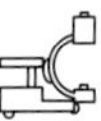

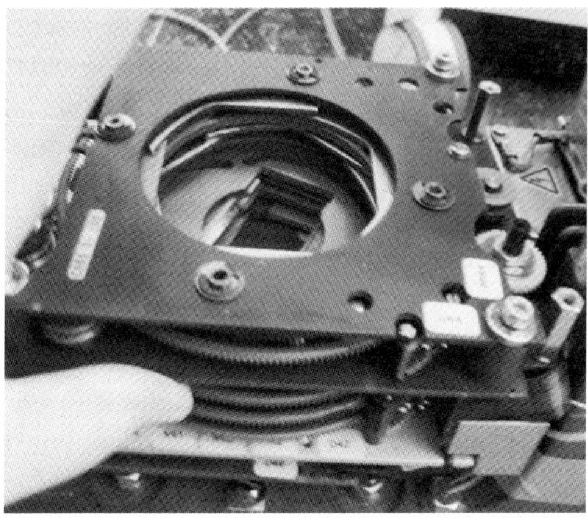

Figure 5.4 Collimators (dose area product meter and casing from Figure 5.1 removed). Iris collimator is on top (retracted), with linear collimators mounted below. Note: linear blades can rotate to change the orientation of beam-shaping.

5.2 **Protection for theatre staff**

Under the Ionizing Radiation (Medical Exposure) Regulations 2000 (IRMER) guidelines, the radiographer is not only responsible for minimizing radiation dose to the patient, but also to the staff present in the theatre while imaging takes place.

When the C-arm is in use, the theatre is a radiation-controlled area. Signs must be in place to inform any staff entering the theatre that it is a controlled environment where ionizing radiation is in use. Some sites may have a 'radiation-controlled area' warning on light-boxes outside entrances to the theatre, while others may have signs (stating that X-rays are in use) that can be attached to the entrances. Be aware that some theatre staff may not regularly work in radiation-controlled areas, and so may be unfamiliar with the rules and precautions in place. As such, it is a good idea to watch out for people entering the theatre during the procedure, and to check whether they are wearing protection before exposure.

Lead (or lead equivalent) protection should be available for all staff, typically in the form of Pb-equivalent aprons. These should fit well and cover down to the knees. They should also be stored correctly when not in use and regularly checked for any defects in the shielding that will allow radiation through. It is often a good idea to have them placed outside the theatre by the entrances (or in the scrub room), so that staff can put them on before entering.

There appears to be a strong link between long-term Pb-equivalent apron usage and associated orthopaedic problems (such as pain in joints and symptoms of spinal problems) (Klein et al. 2009). Some radiologists who wear aprons for a significant amount of time have reported severe back pain, causing them to have to take time off. Some staff may be reluctant to wear them. Most aprons now are designed to share the weight between the wearers' shoulders and hips, by having a separate belt worn around the hips. These can take weight off the wearers' shoulders and back, and should be used whenever available. Lightweight lead-equivalent aprons, which use a combination of lighter materials to offer equivalent protection as a Pb apron, have also become more widely available. These materials can be significantly lighter than lead while offering the same level of protection, and so can be more comfortable to wear for extended periods. Pb-free materials can also be disposed of more easily when the apron has reached the end of its useful life, and may be more resistant to damage and cracking than lead rubber.

Some aprons are designed with very little material on the back to reduce weight. These correspondingly give much less protection when the wearer is facing away from the X-ray source, and so the radiographer should make staff aware of this when they are used. Skirt- and waistcoat-style two-piece aprons are also available, and they can transfer much of their weight to the wearers' hips rather than having the entire weight hanging from the shoulders. These designs may help lessen strain on the wearers' backs.

Remember also that Pb-equivalent aprons can act as reservoirs for infection, and so should be thoroughly cleaned on a regular basis. This is especially important after performing imaging on patients with active infections (Boyle and Strudwick 2010).

Floor- or ceiling-mounted lead shielding is available for general theatres, although these are typically more common in angiography and interventional suites. These systems can have a much thicker lead-equivalence and greater area of protection than aprons, as their weight is far less of a limiting factor. As such, when used properly, they can give much greater protection than an apron. Lead-glass windows can be used to protect the face and neck of surgeons while allowing them to see what they are doing. These units may not be used in place of a Pb-equivalent apron, however, as they do not cover the abdomen and thighs. As such, they are normally used as supplementary protection during high-exposure procedures. Some mobile shields may give

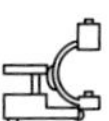

full-length coverage, and so can be used in place of an apron. However, they do not move with a person's body in the same manner as a Pb-equivalent apron does. Hence, if they are used for circulating staff, radiographers must ensure that the staff are behind them whenever imaging is taking place. As such, using such mobile shields can be impractical and may delay imaging.

For cases where imaging was not planned in advance but has become necessary, the scrubbed members of the surgical team may not be wearing any Pb protection under their sterile gowns. To avoid them having to re-gown, some sites may mount a Pb apron on a drip stand or similar and use that as a mobile barrier (often with a sterile gown draped around it) (Lee et al. 2009). This technique is obviously not ideal, as it combines the difficulties of using mobile lead shields with the thinner shielding and reduced coverage of an apron. While this technique is not ideal, it may be the most practical solution if a brief moment of unplanned imaging is required. Having unprotected persons stand behind members of staff who are wearing aprons while imaging occurs puts the responsibility of radiation protection on the aproned members of staff rather than the individuals themselves, and must be avoided. If the case is going to involve long periods of screening, it is normally better for the surgical team to de-gown, put on aprons, and re-scrub. Similarly, it is important to avoid exposing when the surgeons' hands are in the primary beam to avoid dose to the surgeons.

Reduction of exposure to the patient is obviously one of the best ways to reduce radiation dose to the theatre staff, as primary scattered radiation from the patient is the greatest source of dose to theatre staff. Other sources of dose to theatre staff include secondary scatter (radiation backscatter from items in the beam path, including the receptor head) and leakage from the X-ray tube housing. As a rule, any technique that reduces exposure to the patient will also reduce the amount of scatter reaching theatre personnel (Schueler et al. 2006). Collimation of the beam reduces the volume of tissue irradiated, and so can reduce scattered dose to the surgeon and other team members. This can be especially important when imaging larger areas of the patient (e.g. the abdomen, as opposed to the wrist), as thicker regions of tissue will produce more scatter (Brateman 1999) (Figure 5.5).

Involuntary exposure can be avoided by switching off the X-ray circuit whenever it is not in use by turning the key to the 'off' position. If the C-arm is to be left unattended for any length of time, the key should also be removed. This prevents the possibility of unintentional exposures or the use of the machine by untrained persons.

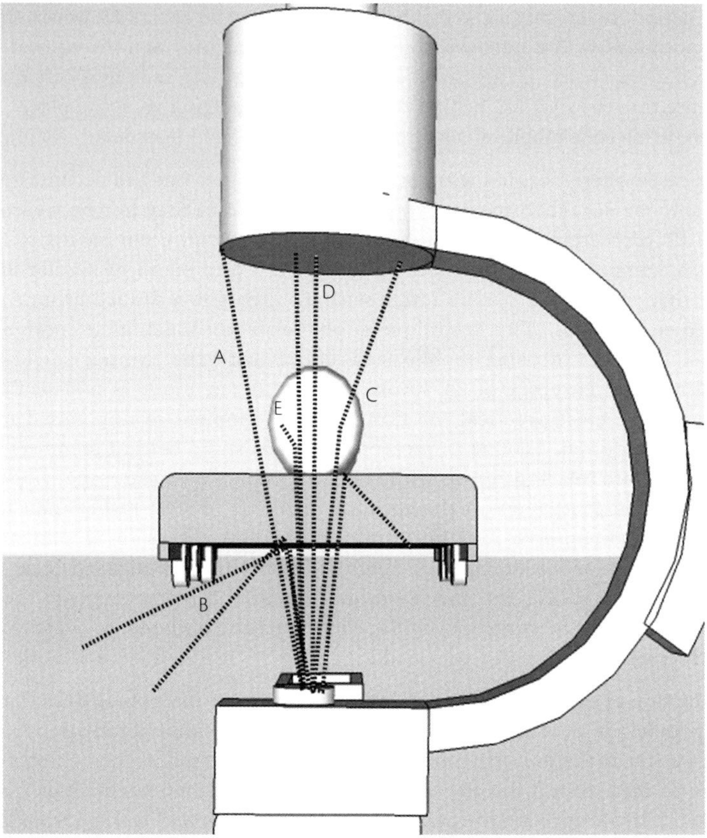

Figure 5.5 Scatter examples. (a) Incident beam not attenuated by patient. (b) Backscatter. (c) Scattered incident beam that will degrade image quality. (d) Incident beam generating image. (e) Internally scattered and absorbed radiation.

It is advisable to remember that it is a requirement for all staff to be using appropriate protection when X-rays are being used, and radiographers are well within their rights to refuse to perform an exposure if staff are not protected.

References

Boyle, H. and Strudwick, R. M. 'Do Lead Rubber Aprons Pose an Infection Risk?', *Radiography*, 16/4 (2010), 297–303.

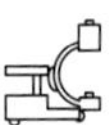

Brateman, L. 'The AAPM/RSNA Physics Tutorial for Residents—Radiation Safety Considerations for Diagnostic Radiology Personnel', *Radiographics: A Review Publication of the Radiological Society of North America, Inc*, 19/4 (1999), 1037–55.

Klein, L., Miller, D., Balter, S., Laskey, W., Haines, D., Norbash, A., Mauro, M., and Goldstein, J. 'Occupational Health Hazards in the Interventional Laboratory: Time for a Safer Environment', *Radiology*, 250/2 (2009), 538–44.

Lee, P., Shanbhag, V., and Iorwerth, A. 'A Simple Technique for Intra-Operative Radiation Protection in Trauma and Orthopaedic Procedures', *Acta Orthopaedica Belgica*, 75/1 (2009), 119–21.

Parry, R. A., Glaze, S. A., and Archer, B. R. 'The AAPM/RSNA Physics Tutorial for Residents—Typical Patient Radiation Doses in Diagnostic Radiology', *Radiographics*, 19/5 (1999), 1289–302.

Schueler, B. A., Vrieze, T. J., Bjarnason, H., and Stanson, A. W. 'An Investigation of Operator Exposure in Interventional Radiology', *Radiographics*, 26/5 (2006), 1533–41.

6

Working in theatre

Theatre practice involves working with staff from many other professions in a collaborative situation, in an environment that includes many factors (such as infection control or other equipment) that are not present or would differ in the X-ray department. As such, it can be an intimidating and unfamiliar place for newly qualified staff, especially when working without assistance for the first time. It is important to try and gain as much familiarity with the theatre environment before working as the lone radiographer in the department. However, there are some basic guidelines that, if followed, should help avoid most potential issues. A short overview of these will be presented here.

6.1 Theatre layout

Most operating theatres consist of a main room where the operation will take place, with a separate anaesthetic room for the induction of anaesthesia. Most theatres have two or three entrances—consisting of a main entrance (for patients and equipment), an anaesthetic room entrance (for moving the anaesthetized patient from the anaesthetic room to the theatre), and an entrance to the clean area or sluices.

The main theatre doors should not be used while a case is underway (this is especially relevant for open orthopaedic cases) unless absolutely necessary. However, it is imperative that the anaesthetic room entrance not be used (nor the anaesthetic staff interrupted) during the induction of anaesthesia, except in an emergency. If the patient is already in the theatre, it is typically best to use the anaesthetic room entrance unless the anaesthetic room is in use with another patient.

Another entrance will connect the theatre with the stock rooms, sluice, or other sections of the theatre block (such as a circulating corridor). This is often used as an entry and exit for staff while a case is underway, and the radiographer should be aware of it in case any staff member enters without protection while imaging is occurring.

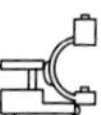

Finally, there is typically an area for staff to scrub up and put on sterile gowns. This is often separated from the main theatre to avoid splashing or contamination.

Most theatres use a system of ventilation where the pressure inside the theatre blows air out through a series of vents into the surrounding rooms. This prevents airborne contaminants from flowing into the theatre where they may contaminate sterile equipment or wounds. Orthopaedic theatres may often feature an ultraclean air system over the centre of the main theatre. This system pumps in highly purified air into the centre of the room over the patient and ensures that the sterile field is shielded from airborne contaminants. It is important to avoid striking the hood of this system with any equipment and to be aware of the area covered by it.

6.2 **Infection control**

Before entering the theatre area, it is necessary to change into appropriate clothing, consisting of clean 'scrubs', hair net or cap that covers all hair, and theatre shoes. This prevents cross-contamination from outside sources of infection. The shoes, in particular, should offer protection from spilled fluids and sharps and be well-fitting and comfortable. As such, while most areas will provide scrubs in a variety of sizes for staff, it can be a good idea to obtain your own theatre shoes to ensure a good fit. A mask is often also necessary, especially in orthopaedics. Most masks feature a metal strip in them that can be moulded around the bridge of the nose. This can help prevent glasses from steaming up while wearing a mask. Some cases will require specialized safety equipment (such as protective tinted glasses if lasers are being used), and these should be available at the start of the case.

Staff must be aware of the sterile fields during a procedure. These will include the regions over and around the patient, the surgical equipment in use and surfaces on which they are kept, and the scrubbed staff.

Items in theatre can be categorized as either sterile or nonsterile. Sterile items are rendered nonsterile if they are touched by any nonsterile item. Once this happens, they must be discarded or replaced. If you see any sterile item (including the surgical teams' gowns and gloves) become contaminated, inform the team immediately to prevent either further items from becoming contaminated or risking infection of the patient's operation site. One must remember that only sterile items can come into contact with other sterile items (Figure 6.1).

Any item of equipment that is going to be in proximity to the patient or other sterile fields may also be covered in a sterile drape to avoid contaminating

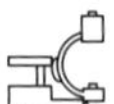

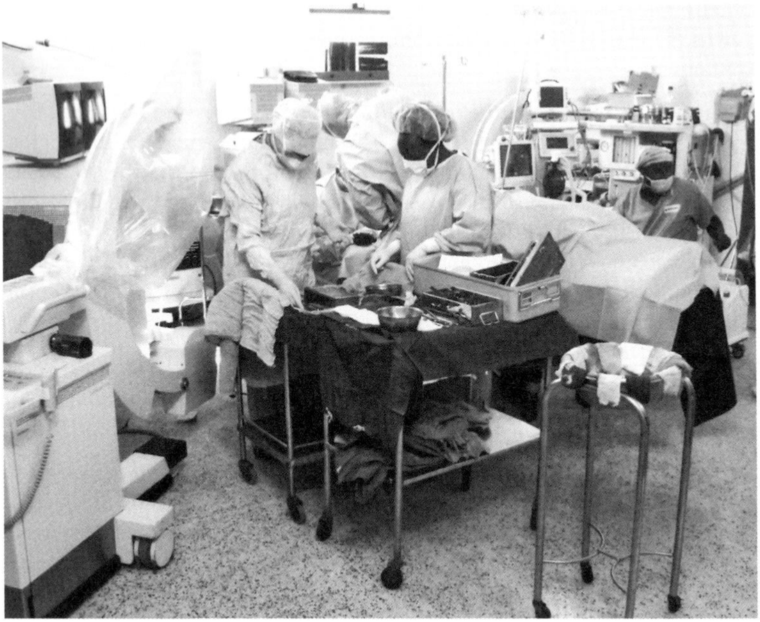

Figure 6.1 Theatre with case underway. Note sterile drape covering II head, staff with sterile gowns. Also note bowl in foreground for used swabs. These will be counted at the end of the case to ensure all consumable items are accounted for.

the fields. This typically includes the receptor for the C-arm. These drapes come in a variety of types and shapes, but all act as a barrier that prevents the nonsterile C-arm receptor from contaminating the sterile fields, while protecting the C-arm from contaminants, including bodily fluids, when it is around the incision sites.

The sterile drape will be placed over the C-arm receptor by one of the scrubbed staff, so as not to contaminate the sterility of the outside of the drape. It is sometimes possible for the radiographer to adjust the drape from inside (where it is in contact with the C-arm and so is already desterilized) if necessary and the radiographer is confident of doing this safely. However, the outside of the drape must *not* be touched by any item that itself is not sterile. If this does happen, inform the theatre team and ask for a replacement drape to be placed on the receptor. If you have any doubt about the sterility of the

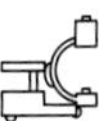

C-arm drape (or any other sterile item), it is your duty to inform the team, so that it can be replaced.

Items used throughout the case may become contaminated with blood or tissues from the patient. It is important for staff to protect themselves from the risks of contact with these. As such, any contaminated item must be handled with gloves (sterile or nonsterile as appropriate). Be especially aware of sharp items that are in use within the theatre. *These can break the skin of staff and risk transferring contaminants into the staff members' bodies. Any sharps injury to any member of staff (including the radiographer) must be reported to the theatre team **immediately**.* It is the duty of all staff to be aware of the sharps injury protocol in use at their site.

If there is risk of splashing, masks and eye protection should also be worn. All theatres should have emergency eyewash available for use in case of contaminants entering the eyes. Any such splash contamination to the eyes should be treated as a sharps injury.

6.3 Entering the theatre

Ensure the C-arm is available and clean before bringing it into the theatre. It should be cleaned after each case, especially where blood or other contaminants are present, or if it has been used with a patient who may have a communicable infection. If there is any dirt or residue from previous cases present on it, clean it again before bringing it in. It is also a good idea to inform any other theatres that have cases requiring X-rays about where you are working and roughly how long the case may take, to update them if delays occur, and to notify them if other radiographers and C-arms are available at the time. Informing the X-ray department about what is happening allows cases and resources to be properly coordinated, and helps avoid delays or situations where more imaging cases are scheduled to take place than the number of available radiographers.

To allow easier setting up of the equipment, the C-arm should be brought into the theatre before the case begins. This also allows the radiographer to check the details of the procedure, enter all patient details into the C-arm system, and introduce themselves to theatre staff and discuss any issues or questions they may have. This is also a good time to check for convenient power outlets and picture archiving and communication system (PACS) network points for the C-arm equipment. Typically, according to the WHO surgical checklist, all theatre staff should introduce themselves and their roles at the start of the case. The patient's identity, pregnancy status, and the procedure that has been planned should be checked by all staff members during the second time out.

If it is not possible to bring in the C-arm before the case begins, it may be brought in through the anaesthetic room doors once the case is underway (assuming that there is no patient in the anaesthetic room).

It is worth checking that there are sufficient Pb-equivalent aprons available for all staff, and that everyone is aware that these will need to be worn before X-rays can be used. Any staff who will be wearing sterile gowns will need to put on this protection before gowning up (unless there are Pb-equivalent shields available; see Chapter 5, 'Radiation protection' for more details). Similarly, any pregnant staff should be made aware that X-rays are to be used before imaging takes place. Announcing that an exposure is to take place in the theatre can allow them time to leave the theatre if needed, or take any other necessary precautions. The warning lights or signs outside the theatre indicating that a case using X-rays is underway should also be checked, to warn any staff from entering the theatre mid-case.

6.4 Safe working within the theatre

All staff within the theatre are responsible for the safety of the theatre team and the patient. The operating theatre is an environment with many hazards that are not present (or present to a far smaller degree) in other areas of the hospital. This includes the risks of sharps and tissue contaminants, as well as other dangers from the equipment in use. This can include electrical risks from diathermy equipment, ionizing radiation from imaging equipment, laser radiation from laser lithotripsy machines, and so on. There are also risks to the patient—including the surgically opened regions of anatomy that can become contaminated or where items can become lost in; monitoring equipment; drains being pulled out; and so on.

Safe working requires a good awareness of what equipment is in use and what risks they may carry, and the ability to communicate any risks or events clearly and confidently to the theatre team.

For cases in which specific protective equipment is required (such as tinted goggles where laser equipment is in use), these should be made available for all staff and used appropriately. If you are uncertain, ask the team what protective equipment you need for the case and when it should be employed.

The equipment and consumables (such as swabs and needles) to be used in the case will be checked and counted by the scrub nurse and circulating staff before the procedure begins. This process will be repeated whenever more

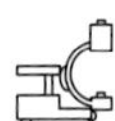

consumables are opened or removed, and at the end of the case. This is to prevent the risk of surgical items being retained within the patient's body by the end of the case. As such, the staff should not be interrupted when performing this task.

All surgical consumables include radio-opaque areas so that they will show up on X-ray. If there are items missing during the final count at the end of the case, the C-arm may be used to help search for the missing items, either by screening the waste bags and drapes, or the regions of the patient's body where the procedure has taken place.

When setting up the C-arm, pay attention to the position of the power cable and the cables connecting the C-arm to the monitors. These may catch on other equipment or stands, especially if the C-arm needs to be repositioned during the case.

Be aware of the sterile fields (such as the equipment trolleys and draped staff) once these have been set up, and avoid touching or letting nonsterile equipment touch these areas and the equipment on them. If a sterile item does get touched by a nonsterile item or member of staff, let the team know, so that it can be replaced.

Be aware of other equipment that may block access to the patient with the C-arm or cause other problems as the case progresses. Many items (such as suction units or diathermy machines) can be moved to more convenient positions if needed; however, it is best to check with the theatre team before doing so.

7

Management of theatre imaging

Generally, multiple operating theatres run simultaneously throughout the course of a day. As such, it is not uncommon for several procedures that require imaging to be underway at the same time. As C-arm systems are expensive, it is unlikely that each theatre will have its own, and so a smaller number of imaging systems will normally be shared across the theatre department. Because of this, it is important for radiographers working in theatre departments to be able to manage their resources effectively and to coordinate with theatre teams to avoid delaying procedures.

When running imaging within theatres the key task is balancing the imaging needs with the available resources. As such, it is vital to know the number of C-arms and staff available, their capacities (e.g. if someone is not capable of doing certain cases, or if some staff require assistance), and the case lists for the day. These should be picked up and checked over at the start of the day for all cases that will require imaging. This step is vital to identify where problems may develop, when extra staff may be required, and when it is best to let staff take breaks or return to the main department if applicable. A good knowledge of procedures will help here; however, if there is any uncertainty, it is important to check with the surgeons performing the case. It is useful to have an estimate for the length of each case, but it is advisable to also be aware that cases may run longer or be delayed in starting.

One must be mindful of any other factors that may affect cases as well—for example, if patients are infectious (which may delay leaving the theatre with equipment after the imaging is completed), or cases that may take longer than originally anticipated (e.g. complex injuries in patients with multiple conditions). Remember that all lists are provisional, and, as such, that things will change throughout the day. Liaising with the theatres performing imaging cases can give advance knowledge of what changes are occurring, and allow the coordinator to inform the theatre teams if there will be a delay in supplying imaging. Theatre cases are a hugely collaborative process between

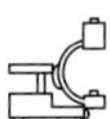

the theatre teams, wards, recovery areas, and other theatres. Each area may have events that may delay or hasten the start or end of a case, and the huge complexity of collaboration and the amount of information that needs to be passed on means that changes to lists and predicted times are almost inevitable.

A good knowledge of C-arm systems is useful (if one is better at certain tasks than others, for example, or has limited image storage, takes a long time to start up or shut down, or has had intermittent problems that may reoccur). Any issues with a C-arm should be recorded, and all staff should be made aware of the issue. Decide if any issue is serious enough to take a machine out of use (e.g. anything affecting radiation output, high-voltage cabling, damage to the II head, or unacceptable loss of image quality).

The radiography team must know how to use the C-arms, to send images and pick-up lists, and to inform others of what is happening with their cases/breaks, and so on.

It is vital to be able to contact the main department (for more staff, if required), and to be contactable by all theatres that will be performing imaging cases. A bleep or phone is useful in this instance. Also useful is a list of the phone numbers of theatres/departments as an aid to coordinating the worklists.

Some radiographers may book all cases onto the local radiological information system (RIS) at the start of the day, and then upload all the case lists onto all the C-arms. This can be useful if there is limited time between cases or limited access to network points. However, any non-performed cases must be marked as such on the RIS at the end of the day, and start/end times should be accurately recorded. Paper records of start/end times, patient doses, and so on can be used throughout the day and entered onto the RIS, but they carry the risk of getting lost or damaged. If used, these must be correctly disposed of at the end of the day, since they carry confidential patient information.

When running the imaging team, it is important to know how the software on the C-arms works, to be able to send images, receive lists, and manually enter and edit patient data on the systems. This is useful for emergency cases or if there are issues with getting to the network points. You should also know how to delete old cases off the C-arms; check doses and screening time; know what format the doses are measured in; and, if this differs from that used on the RIS, how to convert it.

At the end of the day, the radiographers should check that all cases are completed, if there is anything to hand over to the next shift staff (emergency cases, errors with equipment, jobs that need to be done), and that all documentation is completed and all required images sent to the picture archiving and communication system (PACS). The C-arms should also be cleaned and ready for use at short notice.

Consider what can be done if:

- The C-arm is unplugged by accident halfway through a case. (Can you re-enter the exam, or do you have to start a new one? Are the images taken so far saved? How long will it take to restart imaging?)
- The C-arm stops working and cannot function. (Is there another system available? Where is it? How long will it take to get and start using the available system? Is the information on the broken one accessible? Can it be sent to the PACS?)
- An emergency or unplanned case requiring imaging occurs. (When will a C-arm and radiographer be available? Which theatre will it take place in? How will it affect other cases occurring? How long is it likely to last? What is the nature of the case? How will this affect the imaging requirements?)
- A radiographer is taken ill mid-case. (Is he or she okay? What happened? Is there still a risk to other staff? Have team leaders been informed, and the event documented? Who can take over, and how long will it take for them to arrive? How long is the remainder of the procedure? Is there anything that needs handing over?)
- A radiographer is having issues during a case. (Argument with theatre teams, unable to perform required imaging, acting unprofessionally, gone missing, and staff refusing to wear lead protection).

These are rare scenarios; the majority of procedures go smoothly and without incident, thanks to the skill and professionalism of the staff involved.

7.1 Teamwork and professionalism

As a member of the theatres team, it is important to be aware of not only your own role, but also that of the other members of the team. It is important to introduce yourself to the team and to be sure of what procedure is taking place, what will be required, and who will be performing what roles. This should be covered at the start of the procedure, but feel free to ask throughout for clarification if needed.

A professional team works together to complete a task, rather than having individual members working in isolation, and this is as true in surgery as

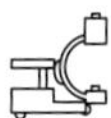

anywhere else. By assisting others in the team when needed, you can help the team, and should be helped in return when required.

Do not rush tasks in an attempt to speed up the case. A slower, considered approach is smoother and often quicker than rushing, especially if things may get overlooked in the process. Similarly, taking a few moments to move around the theatre is better than rushing to get somewhere, desterilizing surfaces or equipment in the process.

If you start to feel dizzy or unwell during a procedure, let the other staff know immediately. Then, stand with your back against the wall, and slowly sit down on the floor. Do not be embarrassed to mention this, and do not try and tough it out! An operating theatre can get very warm, and, combined with the pressures of a long case while wearing Pb-equivalent aprons, the gory nature of some operations can cause people to feel faint. This is quite common, and it is much easier to take 5 min or get another member of staff to cover for you than it is for the rest of the team to deal with someone who has collapsed!

Finally, it is essential to be aware of your own limitations and what you feel comfortable doing. Let other staff know of any difficulties (including staff in other theatres who may be waiting for their own cases), try to plan ahead wherever possible, and try to avoid becoming stressed! Staff (including the radiographer) can become fatigued when working on long cases. It is good to be aware of your own temperament as much as those of others, and, should anyone become irritable, do not take it personally! It is acceptable to let others know if you are getting tired or need a break for whatever reasons. Getting another radiographer to cover for however long is needed is better than souring the atmosphere for want of a break. A calm and respectful approach and a problem-solving attitude will serve you and the team well.

8

Orthopaedics

The majority of cases requiring intra-operative imaging are orthopaedic procedures. These include elective and trauma cases, as well as emergency procedures that may be performed out of regular working hours. They generally involve either repair to the skeleton and joints after injury (e.g. resiting a dislocated joint or aligning and supporting a fractured long bone) or alterations (such as fusion or replacement of a damaged joint, or lengthening of a bone with a growth defect).

The cases discussed here are mostly those covering trauma procedures, although these techniques and positioning may also be employed for elective cases and procedures not covered here. Those covered include procedures such as:

- *Manipulation under anaesthesia* (MUA), the reduction and relocation of structures (such as a joint or fracture site) into the correct anatomical position, performed without opening the surrounding soft tissues, and hence avoiding scarring and infection risk, typically requiring imaging to demonstrate the position of the anatomy.
- *Closed reduction with internal fixation* (CRIF), the reduction and fixation of structures using minimally invasive techniques and internal implants to support the reduction and aid stability, typically requiring imaging to demonstrate the position of the anatomy and implants.
- *Open reduction with internal fixation* (ORIF), the reduction and fixation of structures where incisions are made so that the region can be directly seen and manipulated into position before internal implants are used to support the reduction and aid stability, typically requiring imaging to demonstrate the position of the anatomy and implants outside of the region where they can be seen by the surgeons.
- *External fixation* (Ex Fix), the attachment to bone of a support structure located outside of the patient to support and maintain the reduction of a fracture or apply controlled force to areas of a limb to correct misalignment, typically requiring imaging to demonstrate the position of the anatomy and implantation of attachment pins.

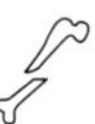

A comprehensive guide to every possible orthopaedic procedure requiring intraoperative imaging would not be practical due to the large number of such procedures and variations involved. Reduction and stabilization of a fractured wrist in a child, for example, may require a different technique to that in an adult, and to that in a more elderly osteoporotic patient, even if the injuries are comparable in all cases. As such, the cases described here should be seen as an overview of the most common procedures and techniques performed, rather than as a definitive guide.

8.1 Manipulation under anaesthesia

If a fracture is displaced, it will need to be manipulated back into alignment if there is to be healing without deformity. In cases where the fracture is non-comminuted and can be reduced to a stable position, an MUA procedure can be performed. These procedures do not require any incisions into the soft tissues, and so minimize the risks of infections and scarring. For these cases, the patient is anaesthetized and the injured area is manipulated back into position by the surgeon by hand. Typically, the region will often then be supported in a cast. Joint relocations are also performed in the same manner. Alternatively, an MUA may be attempted but changed to a CRIF or ORIF procedure if reduction cannot be achieved or maintained, or it may be performed as an emergency case on a more serious fracture before a more invasive procedure can be performed.

8.2 THR relocation

One complication of hip replacement surgery is the risk of dislocation of the prosthesis from the acetabulum. This can be caused via trauma, incorrect positioning or alignment of the implant, or movement of the hip beyond the replacements' stable limits, especially during the first few months after the original replacement surgery. The prosthesis can normally be manipulated back into position with a closed procedure (Valen 2013) (Figure 8.1).

The patient is positioned supine on a radio-lucent table. For relocation of a dislocated hip replacement, patients need to be positioned so that their hips are further down the table than the centre column to allow access for the C-arm. The C-arm is brought in at 90° to the patients' midline, typically from the opposite side to the one under investigation with the tube under-couch, centred over the patients' hip joint. Straight AP images are normally taken at the beginning of the case, and then after manipulation to check for relocation and for any associated damage. The C-arm is moved away during manipulation to allow access to and movement of the hip. Final

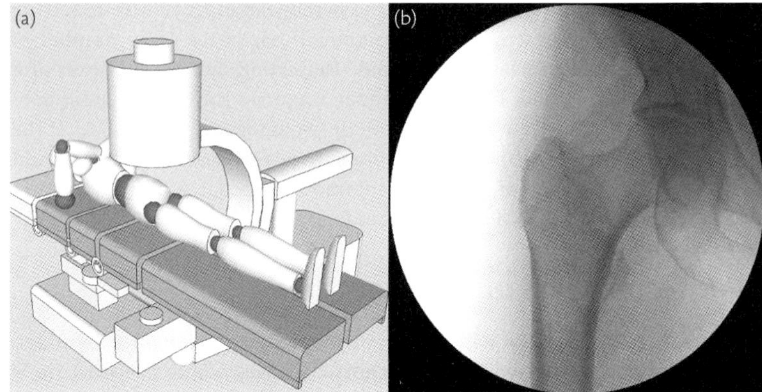

Figure 8.1 Hip positioning. (a) Anteroposterior positioning for the right hip (C-arm brought in from left side). Horizontal beam lateral views will not be required, so the contralateral leg does not need to be moved. (b) Resulting image (no total hip replacement present).

(b) Reproduced courtesy of Radiology Department, Leeds Teaching Hospitals NHS Trust, UK.

AP images demonstrating the relocated hip are saved, as well as some views demonstrating the joint stability if required (e.g. such as internal and external rotation). Views of the end of the hip prosthesis may also be included to check for any periprosthetic damage. All these images should be saved and archived to the picture archiving and communication system (PACS) along with the dose information.

8.3 Shoulder relocation

The shoulder is the most commonly dislocated joint in the body. Typically caused by traumatic injury, with anterior dislocation of the humeral head, dislocations of the shoulder can often be treated without transferring the patient to theatre. However, if several attempts at relocation of the joint have failed, the procedure may be performed in theatres under general anaesthesia. Be aware that there may also be associated injuries from either the original dislocation or from the process of manipulating the joint back into alignment, and these may require further surgical intervention (Marinelli and de Palma 2009) (Figure 8.2).

The patient may be positioned supine or in the beach-chair position. The positioning will affect how the C-arm is brought in over the relevant area. Whichever position is used, to allow the surgeon access, the C-arm should

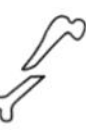

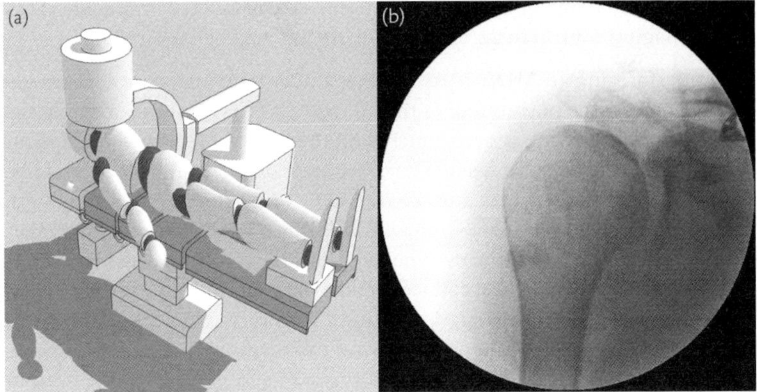

Figure 8.2 Supine anteroposterior (AP) view of shoulder. (a) AP centring of right shoulder joint (supine patient position). Note: the region should not be over the edges of the table, as this can cause beam-occluding artefacts. (b) Resulting image.

(b) Reproduced courtesy of Radiology Department, Leeds Teaching Hospitals NHS Trust, UK.

be positioned such that the receptor is over the shoulder joint and away from the affected side of the patient. See Chapter 9, 'Shoulder and humerus' for further details on C-arm positioning over the shoulder.

The surgeon will then pull on the affected arm and manipulate the humeral head back into position within the glenoid. A straight AP view will then be required, along with some views of the shoulder in internal and external rotation to demonstrate the articular surfaces of the humeral head. An axial or modified axial view may also be performed. If there are any pre-existing surgical implants within the humerus (e.g. a shoulder replacement), then the full length of these will need to be demonstrated to identify any periprosthetic injuries. These images should be saved and archived to the PACS along with the dose information.

8.4 Extremities

Injuries to extremities may often be stable enough to not require any fixation beyond an external splint or casting, but may have some deformity or misalignment at the fracture site. Such injuries may be manipulated under regional anaesthesia with the patient awake, and can be treated in the emergency department. However, for fractures that cannot be reduced in this

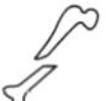

way, or if there is any question about the stability of any reduction, an MUA under imaging control in an orthopaedic theatre will be required.

When performing an MUA of extremities under imaging control, there are two options for the positioning of the C-arm. The first involves rotating the C-arm so that the tube is over-couch, and the affected region of the patient supported on the receptor head. The other position is that the area should be supported on a radio-lucent surface (the table or a suitable extension), with the receptor brought over the limb and withdrawn while manipulation takes place. For many reasons, the over-couch tube and limb supported by the receptor appears superior, as it reduces geometric magnification and unsharpness, removes any unnecessary attenuating structures from the beam path, and ensures minimum OFD, while giving the surgeon much greater access to the limb, reducing ESD to as low as possible, and preventing the need to recentre after moving or adjusting the limb (Figure 8.3).

There are, however, two issues with this position. First, the over-couch tube position means that X-ray backscatter will be reflected upwards towards the thyroid, eyes, and other radiosensitive structures of the surgeons, rather than towards the ground. For this reason, this positioning is not recommended under the Ionizing Radiation (Medical. Exposure) Regulations 2000

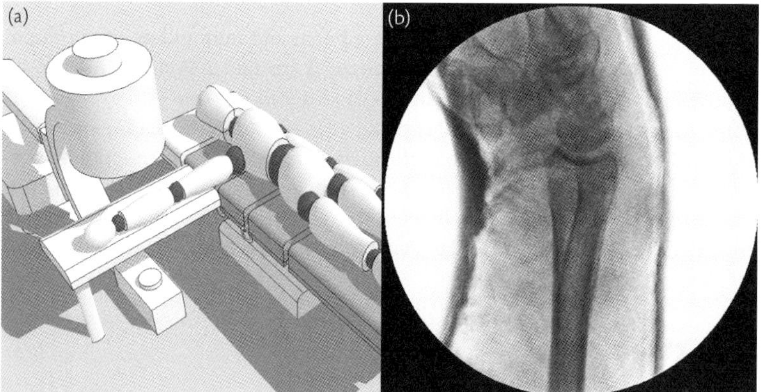

Figure 8.3 Wrist positioning. (a) Standard positioning for right wrist on radio-lucent table extension. The C-arm may also be brought in from the foot-end of the board, depending on how the surgeons will access the limb. Anteroposterior and lateral views are performed by the surgeon rotating the limb. (b) Lateral wrist image. Note the plaster cast in place (dense bands anterior and posterior to the soft tissues).

(b) Reproduced courtesy of Radiology Department, Leeds Teaching Hospitals NHS Trust, UK.

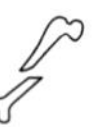

(IRMER) guidelines. The second risk with this positioning is that of damage to the receptor head. A plastic bag over the head can protect it from wet plaster and other detritus, but there is still the risk of other equipment damaging the receptor. It is also worth bearing in mind that C-arm receptors are not typically designed as patient-supporting structures, and damage to the C-arm movement locks may result.

It must be made clear that, whatever the local rules and surgeons' preference, the receptor must ***never*** *be used to support the limb if any surgical hardware such as K-wires are to be implanted.* There is a real risk of sharps piercing the receptor, at best causing the C-arm to need costly repair and desterilizing the item, and at worst risking electrocution of the patient or breaking the vacuum seal in an image intensifier (II), resulting in the intensifier head bursting from the sudden pressure change (Waseem and Kenny 2000).

The under-couch tube position circumvents these problems, but leads to blocking of access to the limb when the C-arm is in place, also resulting in poorer image quality and potentially higher ESD. As such, it is best to follow the departmental rules and surgeons' preference for using the over-couch position, and to only do so (if at all) for cases such as paediatric fractures where the exposure (and hence backscatter) will be low and the image quality is of paramount importance. If used, it is also wise to alert the surgeon to the backscatter risks and take steps to avoid them (moving away from the limb during exposure, use of thyroid shields and Pb glasses, and minimizing exposure time).

If the case is an MUA +/− fixation and the surgeon is insistent on using the receptor as a work surface, it is often possible to start the case with an over-couch tube using the receptor as a surface for the MUA, then to pull back and reset to under-couch orientation (with a table extension attached for support) if internal fixation becomes necessary. This typically occurs during paediatric orthopaedic procedures, and is covered in greater detail in Chapter 17, 'Paediatrics'.

For MUA, the limb will typically be examined under X-ray at the start of the case in multiple planes (AP, lateral, and any others deemed necessary by the surgeon). These will normally be performed by the surgeon manipulating the limb into the desired view. They will then attempt to manipulate the fracture back into position. Imaging may be needed during manipulation, but will definitely be needed to check the reduction afterwards (again, in multiple views to confirm alignment). Post-plaster views may also be needed once the cast is applied to ensure that the reduction has been maintained. Some adjustment to the C-arm position can be useful if the limb is cast in a way that prevents it from being moved freely. For example, an above-elbow

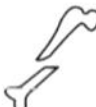

casting of a wrist fracture will prevent the forearm from being rotated for a lateral wrist view, and so the arm will be positioned from the shoulder.

8.5 Joint injection

Injections given directly into joint capsules can be used to administer therapeutic agents into the joint, or to look for damage or injuries to the capsule itself by use of contrast agents. These minimally invasive procedures are very versatile and can allow dynamic and stress-view visualization of joint structures. An injection into the hip is covered in the following text; however, with careful positioning and C-arm approach, they can be adapted to cover most synovial joints in the body.

Patient position

- Supine, with the joint under investigation on a radio-lucent support

C-arm approach

- Centred over the joint under investigation in AP view, at 90° to the limb

Key imaging

- *AP view of joint pre-injection*
- *AP view of joint post-contrast injection*
- *AP/lateral views of joint manipulated by surgeon if required*

Procedure

- The patient is positioned supine on the table with the joint under investigation supported as necessary.
- The region is cleaned and a small drape placed around it. *The C-arm is brought in from the opposite side to the surgeons, and a single image is taken to demonstrate the joint space.*
- A needle is inserted towards the joint. An image may be required to demonstrate the tip within the joint.
- The needle tip position is checked by drawing back some synovial fluid through the needle. *Iodine contrast agent is then injected into the joint space. One or more AP views may be performed to monitor the contrast agent flow into the joint.*

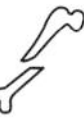

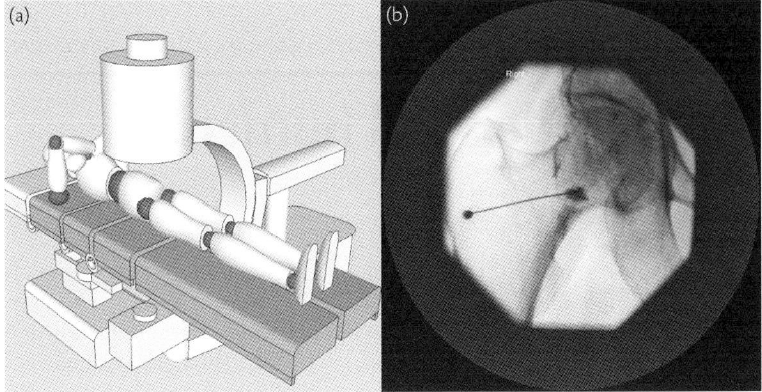

Figure 8.4 Hip injection. (a) Anteroposterior (AP) positioning of right hip. Horizontal beam lateral views are not required, so the contralateral limb is not repositioned. (b) Resulting AP image with needle and contrast visible. Note iris collimation in use. The acetabulum must remain visible.

(b) Reproduced courtesy of Radiology Department, Leeds Teaching Hospitals NHS Trust, UK.

- The joint may be manipulated to demonstrate other aspects of the articular surfaces and joint capsule. *Images should be taken and saved for each of these views when prompted by the surgeon.*
- The needle is removed and a dressing is placed over the injection point. *The saved pre- and post-contrast images should be saved to the PACS with the dose summary* (Figure 8.4).

References

Marinelli, M. and de Palma, L. 'The External Rotation Method for Reduction of Acute Anterior Shoulder Dislocations', *Journal of Orthopaedic Traumatology*, 10/1 (2009), 17–20

Valen, B. 'Dislocation of Hip Prostheses', *Tidsskr Nor Legeforen nr*, 133/11 (2013), 1197–99.

Waseem, M. and Kenny, N. W. 'The Image Intensifier as an Operating Table—a Dangerous Practice', *The Journal of Bone and Joint Surgery*, 82/1 (2000), 95–96.

9

Shoulder and humerus

The shoulder or proximal humerus injury can often be treated conservatively, with sling support and regular monitoring to check healing. However, surgical intervention is sometimes required to ensure correct reduction and functionality of the limb. Due to the location of the shoulder and humerus next to the torso and the relative infrequency of such procedures, they can represent a challenge for the radiographer.

9.1 Open plating of clavicle

Due to the superficial nature of the clavicle, almost all its length can be exposed by the surgeon, and imaging may hence not be required. However, imaging may be indicated due to the severity of the fracture or the surgeons' preference.

Patient position

- Beach-chair position, with the patient in the middle of the table

C-arm approach

- From the head-end of the table along the sagittal plane, with the C-arm rotated away so that the receptor head is parallel to the coronal plane, and centred over and angled parallel to the affected clavicle
- Alternatively, from the opposite side of the patient at 90° to the sagittal plane with the C-arm tilted, so that the receptor head is parallel to the coronal plane, and centred over and angled parallel to the affected clavicle

Key imaging

- *AP/oblique clavicle views for reduction*
- *AP/oblique clavicle views for fit of plate*
- *AP/oblique clavicle views for implant position, reduction, and screw lengths*

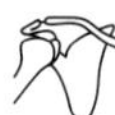

Procedure

- The patient is cleaned and draped. *The C-arm is draped over the receptor, and the fracture site is identified by the AP and oblique clavicle views.*
- The region over the clavicle is opened, and the fracture located. The fracture site is manually reduced and held in place with clamps.
- A plate is selected and placed onto the clavicle once the reduction appears satisfactory. *The surgeon may wish to check the fit of the plate under AP and oblique clavicle views.*
- If the fit of the plate on the bone is not satisfactory, it may be replaced with a different size, or manually bent to better fit the anatomy of the patient. *Once this is done, the fit of the plate can be checked again under AP and oblique clavicle views.*
- Once the surgeon is satisfied with the fit of the plate, it is fixed to the anterior surface of the clavicle with screws. *The C-arm should be withdrawn from over the patient while this occurs to give the surgeon better access.* Imaging to judge the depth of the screws should not normally be required at this point.
- *Depending on the stability of the reduction and placing of the screws, the surgeon may require fresh AP and oblique clavicle views to demonstrate the fracture reduction once the first screws are in place.* The remaining screws are then inserted through the plate into the bone.
- *Final AP and oblique clavicle views are taken to demonstrate the implant, fracture reduction, and screw lengths. These should be saved to the picture archiving and communication system (PACS) with the dose summary* (Figure 9.1).

9.2 Screw fixation of tuberosity fractures

The greater and lesser tuberosity of the humerus are attachment points for the tendons that allow movement at the shoulder joint. Fractures of the greater tuberosity may occur in isolation or in combination with other fractures or dislocation of the shoulder joint, while lesser tuberosity fractures are typically caused by high-energy trauma and very rarely seen in isolation. As such, any fixation applied to them may be in combination with other surgical interventions to the region (such as proximal humeral plating or nailing) for associated injuries. Due to the more common nature of the injury, this section will focus on fractures to the greater tuberosity (Robinson et al. 2009).

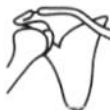

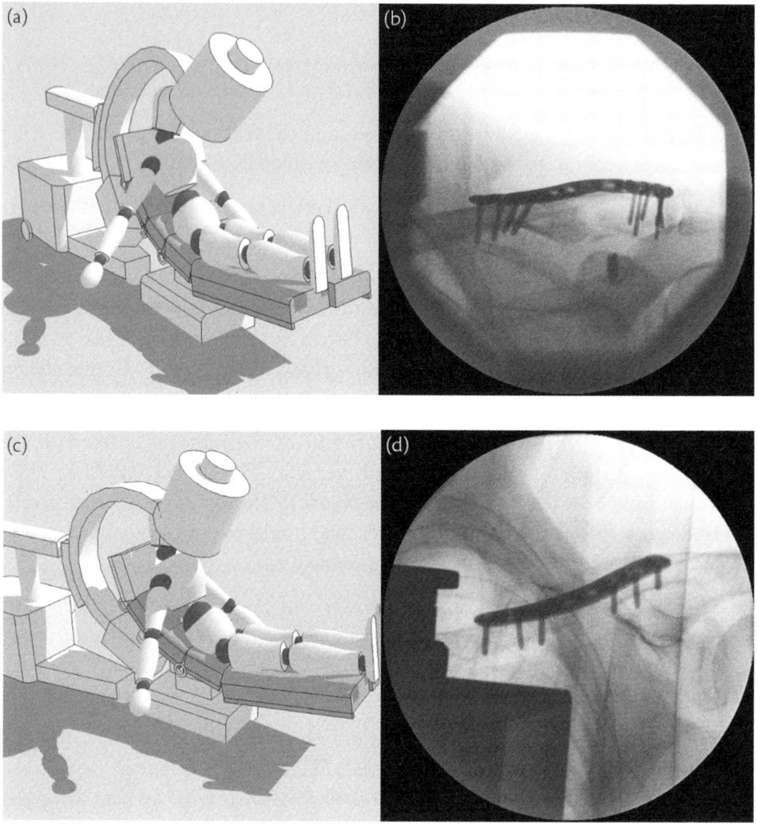

(a) (b) (c) (d)

Figure 9.1 Clavicle plating. (a) Anteroposterior clavicle position. Receptor angled away from patient's head. (b) Resulting image. Note clavicle projected clear from scapula. (c) Angled clavicle view; C-arm rotated to more vertical. (d) Resulting image, with clavicle overlying superior ribs.

(b) and (d) Reproduced courtesy of Radiology Department, Leeds Teaching Hospitals NHS Trust, UK.

Patient position

- Beach-chair position, with the affected limb brought to the side away from the table edge

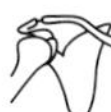

C-arm approach

- From the head-end of the table along the sagittal plane, with the C-arm rotated away so that the receptor head is parallel to the coronal plane, and centred over the affected shoulder
- Alternatively, from the opposite side of the patient at 90° to the sagittal plane with the C-arm tilted so that the receptor head is parallel to the coronal plane, and centred over the affected shoulder

Key imaging

- *AP view with arm rotated for fracture reduction*
- *AP view with arm rotated for insertion of K-wires and screws*
- *AP image parallel to glenoid/axial views for joint space*
- *AP/lateral/axial/Y views for final check of implants and reduction*

Procedure

- The tuberosity is manipulated back into anatomical position, either with the limb closed or with a surgical implement inserted through the lateral aspect of the shoulder. *Imaging of the region is undertaken in the AP view to show the site of the fragment in relation to the humerus* (Figure 9.2).
- Once the fragment is in an acceptable position, a K-wire is driven through the fragment and into the humerus under imaging control as a temporary fixation. *AP views may be taken with the arm rotated to show the path of the K-wire within the humerus, and, if applicable, the position in relation to the articular surfaces* (Figure 9.3).
- Due to the spherical shape of the humeral head, the screws are inserted at various angles so as not to strike each other and to gain as much purchase on the bone as possible. *It is important to identify any penetration of implants through the articular surface of the humeral head as this will compromise the joint space. Angulation of the C-arm so that the central ray is parallel with the glenoid may be required.*
- A cannulated screw is inserted over the K-wire and driven through the fragment into the humerus under imaging control. *Once the screw is in place, its position will be rechecked under imaging as before.* For large or

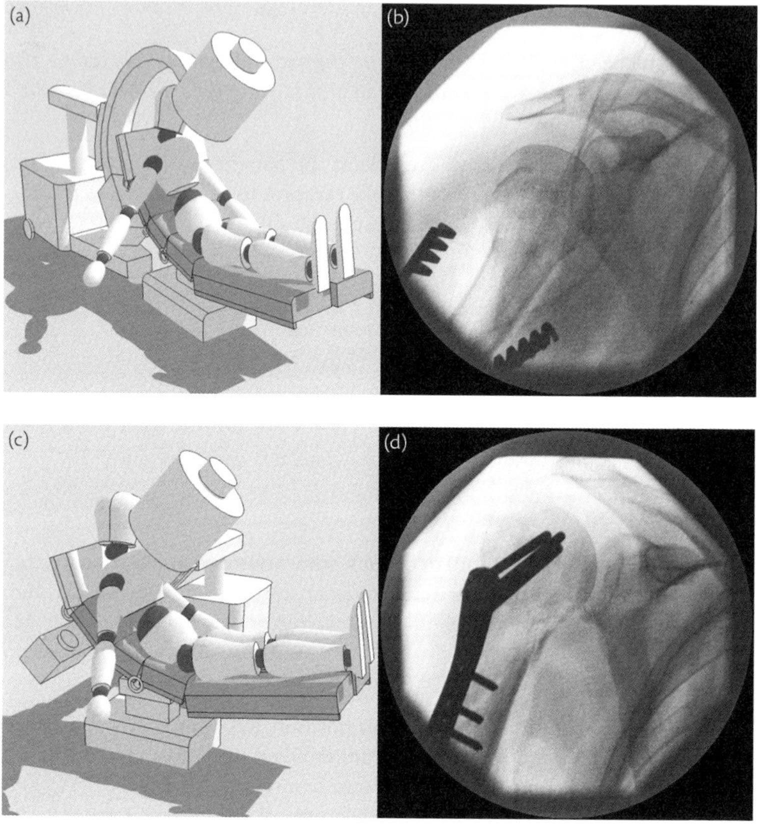

Figure 9.2 Shoulder positioning. (a) Anteroposterior (AP) view of shoulder from overhead approach. Note the tilt of the C-arm, so that receptor is closer to the patient's head. This helps put the glenoid in profile. (b) Resulting image. Humerus is rotated here. (c) Alternate approach to AP of shoulder. (d) AP with humerus in neutral position, proximal plate *in situ*.

(b) and (d) Reproduced courtesy of Radiology Department, Leeds Teaching Hospitals NHS Trust, UK.

unstable fragments, a second screw may also be inserted in the same manner.

- Once all the screws are in satisfactory position, the K-wires and any reduction clamps are removed. *Final AP images are taken with the arm rotated by the surgeon demonstrating the fracture and screw positions. A lateral or axial*

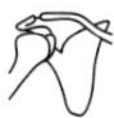

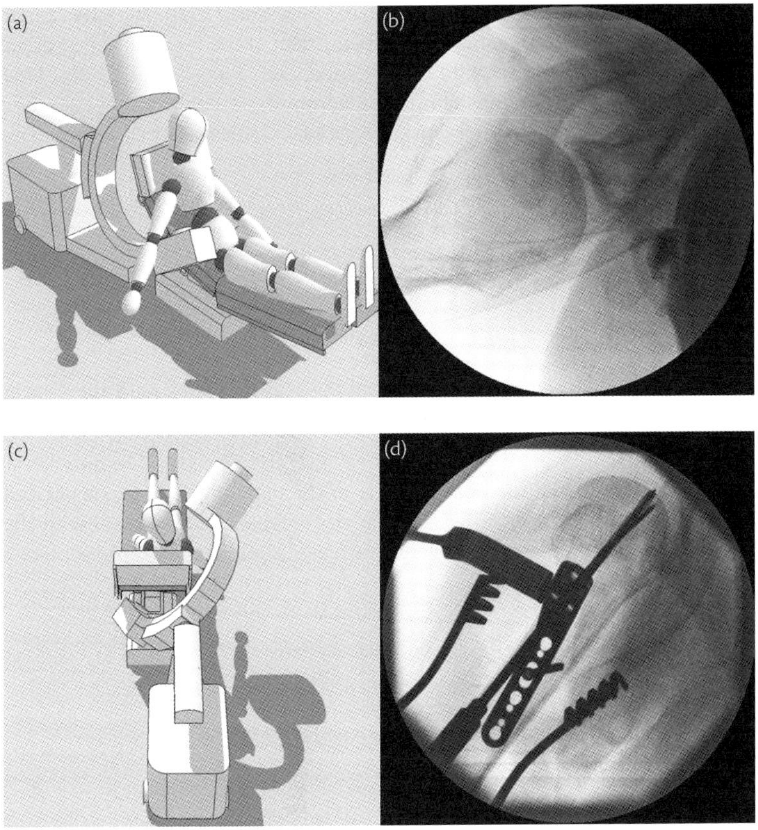

(a) (b) (c) (d)

Figure 9.3 Further shoulder positioning. (a) Axial view from overhead approach. Note: this view is not possible with alterative lateral approach. (b) Resulting axial shoulder image. (c) Lateral scapula/Y view from overhead approach. Note: this view is not possible with alternative lateral approach, and beam direction avoids the table edges. (d) Resulting image showing K-wires in humeral head.

(b) and (d) Reproduced courtesy of Radiology Department, Leeds Teaching Hospitals NHS Trust, UK.

view may also be required. The C-arm can then be withdrawn, and these images must be sent to the PACS along with the dose summary.

9.3 **Proximal humerus plating**

Undisplaced fractures of the proximal humerus often require no surgical intervention, as conservative management can achieve a satisfactory outcome.

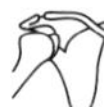

As such, these procedures are less regularly performed than fixation of other regions. However, for patients with displacement at the fracture site or other complications, internal fixation may be indicated (Fakler et al. 2008). Due to the position of the regions of interest, combined with the relative scarcity of such operations, these interventions can be a challenge for radiographers.

Patient position

- Beach-chair position, with the affected limb brought to the side away from the table edge

C-arm approach

- From the head-end of the table along the sagittal plane, with the C-arm rotated away so that the receptor head is parallel to the coronal plane, and centred over the affected shoulder
- Alternatively, from the opposite side of the patient at 90° to the sagittal plane with the C-arm tilted, so that the receptor head is parallel to the coronal plane, and centred over the affected shoulder

Key imaging

- *AP views with arm rotated for fracture reduction*
- *AP views with arm rotated for insertion of K-wires and screws*
- *AP image parallel to glenoid/axial views for joint space*
- *Lateral/Y view for position of plate on humerus*
- *AP/lateral/axial/Y views for final check of implants and reduction*

Procedure

- *The fracture is located using multiple AP views with rotation of the limb by the surgeon.* The fracture is then manipulated into anatomical position by traction and manipulation of the arm. *The C-arm is withdrawn while cleaning and draping takes place.*
- The surgical site is opened and the fracture site located. *Clamps may be used to hold the fracture site in reduction; it is important to be aware of these and to be careful to not compromise the reduction by striking them when moving the C-arm.* K-wires may also be inserted as temporary fixation and as guides for cannulated screws (Figure 9.4).
- A humeral plate is inserted onto the lateral aspect of the humerus to check the fit and positioning around the fracture. *The whole length of the*

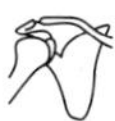

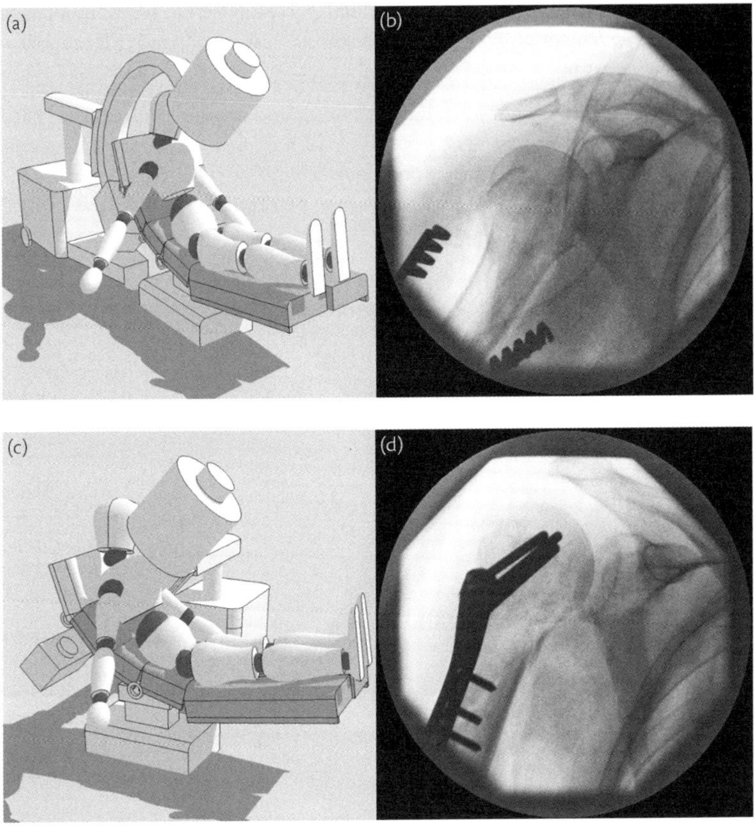

Figure 9.4 Shoulder positioning. (a) Anteroposterior (AP) view of shoulder/humeral head from head-end approach. (b) Resulting AP image (humerus rotated), with tissue retractor in view. (c) Alternate AP approach from contralateral side. (d) Resulting AP image with plate and screws *in situ*.

(b) and (d) Reproduced courtesy of Radiology Department, Leeds Teaching Hospitals NHS Trust, UK.

plate should be demonstrated on AP images, as well as the shoulder joint and acromioclavicular joint. A plate that is too long or positioned too superiorly can strike the acromion when raising the arm, reducing the patients' effective range of movement of the limb. *As such, views covering the range of movement of the humerus may be performed.*

- Once the surgical team is satisfied with the plate and position, it is temporarily fixed to the humerus with K-wires. *Guide holes for screws are drilled into the humeral head through the plate, the positioning of which will be checked by multiple AP views with rotation of the limb to demonstrate the humeral head* (Figure 9.5).

- Due to the spherical shape of the humeral head, the screws are inserted at various angles so as not to strike each other and to gain as much purchase on the bone as possible. *It is important to identify any penetration of implants through the articular surface of the humeral head as this will compromise the joint space.* Angulation of the C-arm may be required, so that the central ray is parallel with the glenoid.

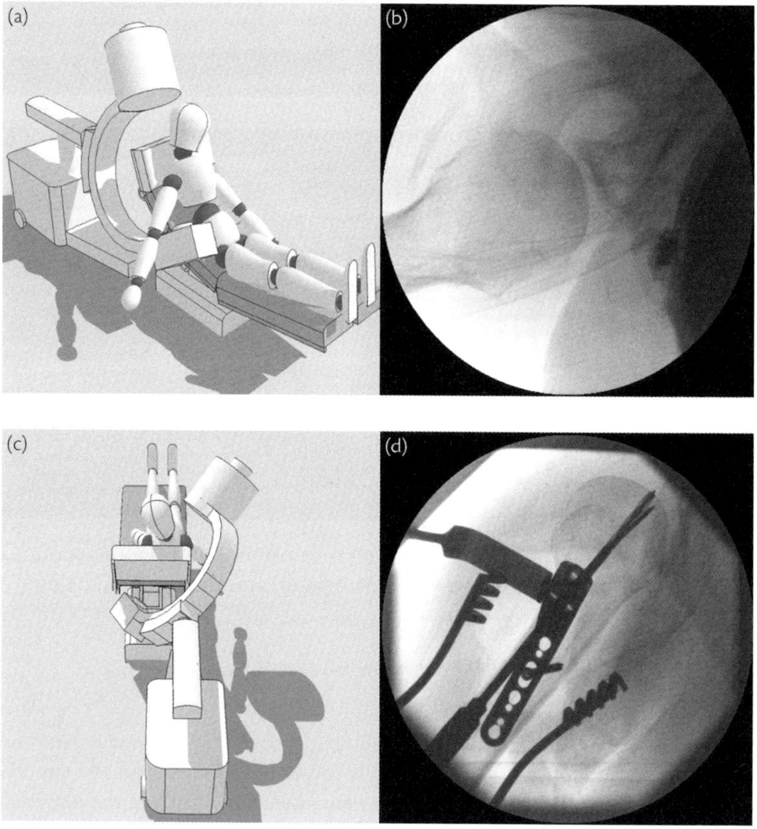

(a) (b)

(c) (d)

Figure 9.5 Further positioning for shoulder plating. (a) Axial view of shoulder (only possible from head-end approach (b) Resulting Axial image (c) Modified Y-view/Lateral scapula view (d) Resulting image demonstrating lateral humerus and plate attached.
(b) and (d) Reproduced courtesy of Radiology Department, Leeds Teaching Hospitals NHS Trust, UK

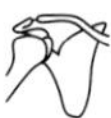

- A lateral humerus/Y-view may also be required to demonstrate the plate position on the humerus. *When using this view, be aware of any reduction aids or drill guides still attached to the patient.*
- The plate is then secured to the humeral head with screws, and distal screws are placed through the plate into the humeral shaft. *The path and depth of the distal screws may be checked using an AP view showing the distal aspect of the plate.*
- The temporary supports of the fracture and plate (clamps, K-wires) are removed. *The final positioning of the plate and fracture is again checked under multiple AP and lateral views, which are then saved to the PACS along with the dose summary.*

9.4 **Humeral shaft plating**

Humeral plates may be used where surgical fixation of a humeral shaft fracture is required and intramedullary (IM) nailing is infeasible or contraindicated—for example, fractures to the proximal or distal regions of the humerus or those with associated injuries to the arm, such as nerve or vascular entrapment, that require intervention to release the structures.

The positioning of the patient will depend on the position of the fracture, intended placement of the plate, and the surgeons' preference. There are three surfaces of the humerus to which a plate may be applied, these being the anterolateral, medial, and posterior.

Patient position

- Supine, with the arm supported on a radio-lucent support (for anterolateral or medial plating)
- Beach-chair position, with the affected limb brought to the side away from the table edge (for anterolateral plating)
- Prone, with the affected arm abducted and supported on a radio-lucent board, with the elbow flexed to the floor (for posterior plating)
- Lateral decubitus position with the affected arm on top and extended anteriorly to the patient, the elbow flexed over a radio-lucent support, and the forearm allowed to hang downwards (for posterior plating)

C-arm approach (beach-chair)

- From the head-end of the table along the sagittal plane, with the C-arm rotated away so that the receptor head is parallel to the coronal plane, and centred over the affected shoulder

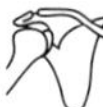

- Alternatively, from the opposite side of the patient at 90° to the sagittal plane with the C-arm tilted so that the receptor head is parallel to the coronal plane, and centred over the affected shoulder

C-arm approach (prone, decubitus, supine)

- From the head or foot-end of the table and parallel with the patient's torso, with the C-arm centred over the midshaft of the humerus

Key imaging

- *AP/lateral views for reduction*
- *AP/lateral views for insertion of plate if minimally invasive technique used*
- *Lateral view for screw depth and position*

Procedure

- A minimally invasive approach will require imaging throughout to view the plate along the humerus as it is inserted. In this technique, relatively small incisions are made above and below the fracture site, and the plate is inserted along the humerus until it is in a good position. *Minimally invasive techniques are only applicable when the plate is to be positioned along the anterolateral surface of the humerus.*
- Alternatively, an open approach can be used, where the limb is opened along the entire length of the plate. Less imaging will be required for this technique, as the surgeon can see the plate in relation to the humerus directly. *This technique can be used for attaching a plate to any of the surfaces of the humerus, and where there are complications to the injury (such as entrapment of the radial nerve at the fracture site) that require intervention* (Figure 9.6).
- The patient is positioned, and the fracture is manually reduced into anatomical position. *Images in AP and lateral views of the fracture site will be required, and views of the proximal and distal humerus may also be needed to ensure the limb is aligned and not rotated at the fracture.*
- An external reduction aid may be attached to the bone in cases of comminuted fractures or where the reduction is very unstable. If used, it is important to avoid striking this with the C-arm while performing imaging.
- The plate to be used is selected, and may be measured against the humerus under imaging to ensure it is a good length relative to the position of the fracture site. The plate may also be contoured to better fit the humerus.
- The region of the patient is then cleaned and draped, and the limb is opened. In minimally invasive procedures, a small incision is made

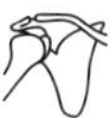

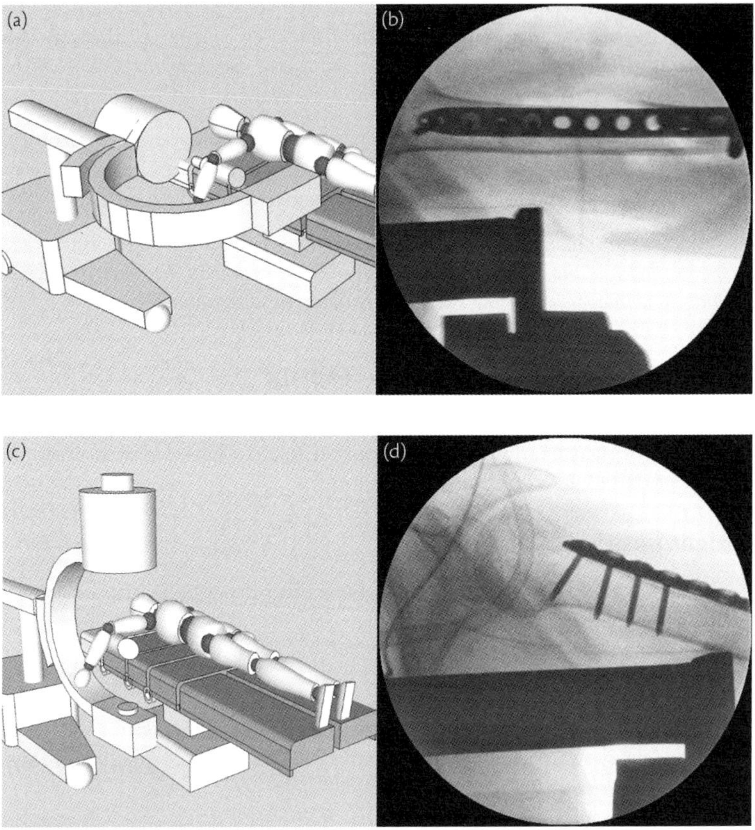

(a) (b) (c) (d)

Figure 9.6 Prone humeral plating. (a) Lateral approach for proximal humerus (Be aware of elbow in relation to the C-arm!). (b) Resulting image showing plate on humerus. (c) Anteroposterior positioning (prone) for humerus. (d) Resulting image.

(b) and (d) Reproduced courtesy of Radiology Department, Leeds Teaching Hospitals NHS Trust, UK.

proximally and distally to the fracture site. *The plate is then inserted along the bone under imaging control.* The fracture site will need to be checked as the plate crosses it to ensure the reduction is maintained and the plate remains aligned on the humerus. *Once the plate appears in a satisfactory position on the AP view, a lateral view may also be performed to ensure the position of the plate on the humeral surface.*

- For more open procedures, the tissues are opened along the shaft of the humerus and the plate is placed against the bone across the fracture site.

- Once the position of the plate and limb appear satisfactory both on imaging and appearance of the limb, the first screw is inserted through the plate into the bone for fixation. *The path and depth of the screw will be checked under imaging, in a view lateral to the plate.*
- Once this provisional fixation of the plate to the limb appears satisfactory, more screws are inserted in the same manner (at least the two screws proximal and distal to the fracture site) to give definitive fixation.
- *Once the fixation is complete, AP and lateral views are taken to demonstrate the entire length of the plate and fracture site. The C-arm can then be withdrawn, and these images sent to the PACS along with the dose summary.*

9.5 Humerus antegrade IM nailing

Fractures of the humerus may in isolation be managed conservatively. However, surgical fixation may be required (e.g. in patients with multiple trauma or pathological fractures of the limb).

Patient position

- Beach-chair position, with the affected limb brought to the side away from the table edge

C-arm approach

- From the head-end of the table along the sagittal plane, with the C-arm rotated away so that the receptor head is parallel to the coronal plane, and centred over the affected shoulder
- Alternatively, from the opposite side of the patient at 90° to the sagittal plane with the C-arm tilted, so that the receptor head is parallel to the coronal plane, and centred over the affected shoulder

Key imaging

- *AP/lateral views for preliminary reduction and measurements*
- *AP view of shoulder for entry point*
- *AP view of humerus for insertion of nail*
- *AP/oblique/lateral views of shoulder for proximal locking screws*
- *AP/lateral views of elbow for distal locking*
- *AP/lateral views of humerus for end-cap, reduction, and fracture site*

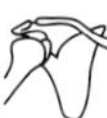

Procedure

- A provisional reduction is made by manually manipulating the distal humerus so that the fracture is in adequate alignment. *The position of the fracture site may then be checked in AP and lateral views (performed by rotating the humerus) to ensure reduction at the site* (Figure 9.7).
- Measurements can be made with a radiographic ruler to determine the length and diameter of the nail to be implanted. *The end of the ruler is aligned with the insertion site of the nail at the humeral head in the AP view. The C-arm is then moved to demonstrate the distal humerus, and another AP view taken.* The length of the nail to be implanted can then be measured along the medullary canal. *If the ruler is placed over the humerus, the width markers can also be used to gauge the width of the medullary canal at its narrowest point, and so give the maximum diameter of nail that can be used.*
- The insertion site at the head of the humerus is opened. *An AP view of the head may be useful as the bone is opened and the insertion hole widened to allow insertion of the nail.* Once the insertion point is satisfactory, the nail is inserted on the positioning jig into the proximal humerus.
- *An AP view of the fracture site is then required as the nail is advanced.* Once the nail reaches the fracture site, it is progressed across the fracture into the distal section. *Manipulation of the lower end of the limb may be required to align the medullary canal with the nail. Once the nail has crossed into the distal segment on the AP view, a lateral view will be required to ensure the nail is fully within the canal.* The nail is then advanced down towards the condyles.
- The proximal locking screws are inserted laterally through the humeral head. *An AP view of the region is required as the guide hole is drilled through the lateral border of the humerus and locking holes of the nail.* The depth of the drill is checked under AP views to prevent it from crossing into the glenohumeral joint.
- Once the depth is satisfactory, the length of the screw hole is measured, and the appropriate-length screw is inserted. *The position of this screw must be checked under several views, including an AP and additional views performed either by rotating the humerus to demonstrate the articular surfaces, or an axial view if possible.* The process is then repeated for the second screw. Views showing both the proximal locking screws in position should be saved for archiving.
- *Before the distal locking screws are inserted, the reduction and alignment at the fracture site may be rechecked under AP and lateral views to identify any adjustments that need to be made to the positioning before continuing.*

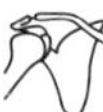

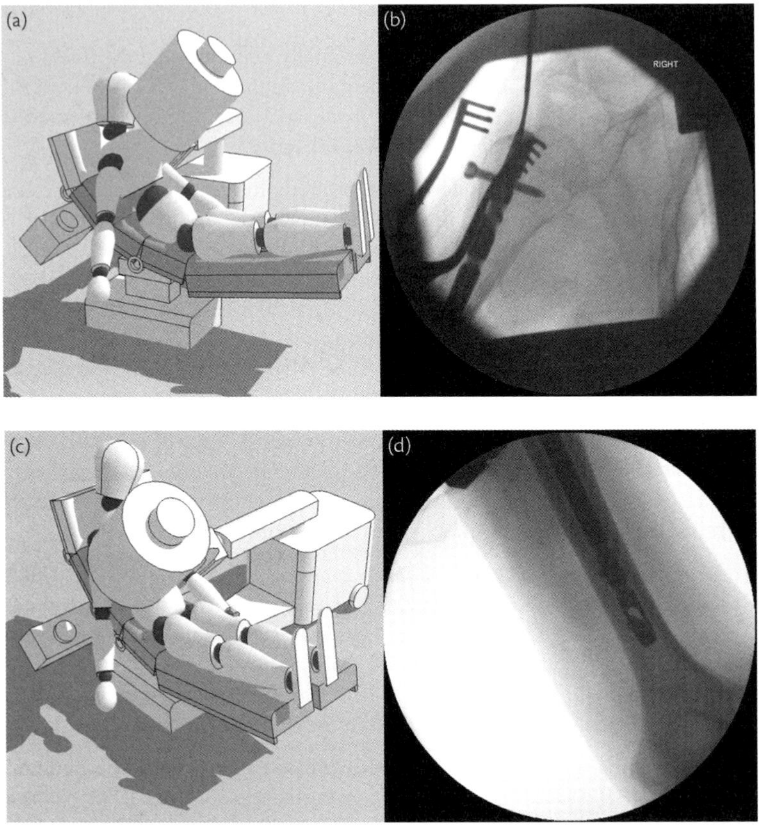

Figure 9.7 Beach-chair approach for humeral nail. (a) Anteroposterior (AP) view of shoulder in beach-chair position. (b) Resulting image showing nail inserted. (c) AP of elbow in beach-chair position. (d) Resulting image showing distal locking screws.
(b) and (d) Reproduced courtesy of Radiology Department, Leeds Teaching Hospitals NHS Trust, UK.

- The distal screws are inserted freehand through the anterior surface of the humerus. *The C-arm is repositioned so that it is centred over the distal locking screws in the AP position.* The position of the locking hole is then found under AP view, and the surrounding soft tissues opened. A drill is then placed onto the surface of the humerus and its position checked, so that the tip is directly over the locking hole.
- Once the positioning of the drill is correct, the surgeon will drill a guide hole for the screw through the humerus and locking hole. The depth

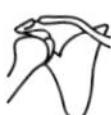

of the hole is then measured, and an appropriate-sized locking screw is inserted into the guide hole and through the nail. *This is then checked in AP and lateral views, before the second screw is inserted in the same manner. Views showing both the distal locking screws in position should be saved for archiving.*

- *The fracture site may be rechecked under AP and lateral views before the tissues are closed.* These views should be saved for archiving.
- The positioning jig is then removed from the end of the nail, and an end-cap is inserted onto the proximal section of the nail where the jig was previously attached. *An AP of the humeral head with the end-cap in place should also be performed to show the final position of the nail. This image, along with multiple views of the fracture site and both proximal and distal screws, should be saved to the PACS along with the dose information.*

9.6 Humerus retrograde IM nailing

For fractures of the proximal humerus, it may not be practical to insert an IM nail via the antegrade approach. In such cases, a retrograde approach from the distal humerus may be used.

Patient position

- Prone, with the affected arm abducted and supported on a radio-lucent board, with the elbow flexed to the floor

C-arm approach

- At 90° to the shaft of the humerus from the lateral side, with the receptor centred over the humerus

Key imaging

- *AP/lateral views for reduction of fracture site*
- *AP/lateral views of distal humerus for nail insertion*
- *AP/lateral views of fracture site for nail insertion*
- *AP/lateral views of distal humerus for locking screw insertion*
- *AP/lateral views of proximal humerus for locking screw insertion*
- *AP/lateral views of fracture site for compression reduction (if used)*
- *AP/lateral views of distal humerus for end-cap*

Procedure

- A provisional reduction is made by manually manipulating the distal humerus so that the fracture is in adequate alignment. *The position of the fracture site may then be checked in AP and lateral views to ensure reduction at the site.* The lateral view may be performed by rotating the C-arm to the horizontal beam lateral (HBL) position.
- Measurements are made with a radiographic ruler to determine the length and diameter of the nail to be implanted. *The end of the ruler is aligned with the insertion site of the nail by the condyles in the AP view.* Then the C-arm is moved medially to demonstrate the humeral head. *The length of the nail to be implanted can then be measured along the medullary canal from the AP view of the humeral head.* If the ruler is placed over the humerus, the width markers can also be used to gauge the width of the medullary canal at its narrowest point and so give the maximum diameter of nail that can be used (Figure 9.8).
- The insertion site at the condyles is opened. *An AP view of the head may be used as the bone is opened and the insertion hole widened to allow insertion of the nail.* A lateral view may also be used to show the entrance to the medullary canal and so avoid a steep insertion angle that may block the nail. Once the insertion point is satisfactory, the nail is inserted on the positioning jig into the distal humerus.
- Once the nail reaches the fracture site, it is progressed across the fracture into the proximal section. *An AP view of the fracture site is then required as the nail is advanced.* Manipulation of the limb may be required to align the medullary canal with the nail. *Once the nail has crossed into the proximal segment on the AP view, a lateral view will be required to ensure the nail is fully within the canal.*
- The nail is then advanced down towards the humeral head. Once the end of the nail is in a satisfactory position within the humeral head, the locking screws can be inserted. *AP and lateral views of the distal humerus may be required at this point to ensure that the nail is correctly located and not protruding at the entry point.*
- The distal locking screws are inserted using the positioning jig through the posterior humerus. A guide hole is drilled through the posterior border of the humerus and locking holes of the nail. *The depth of the drill is checked under lateral views to ensure it crosses the anterior humerus and does not protrude into the soft tissues.* Once the depth is satisfactory, the length of the screw hole is measured, and the appropriate-length screw is inserted. The process is then repeated for the second screw.

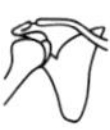

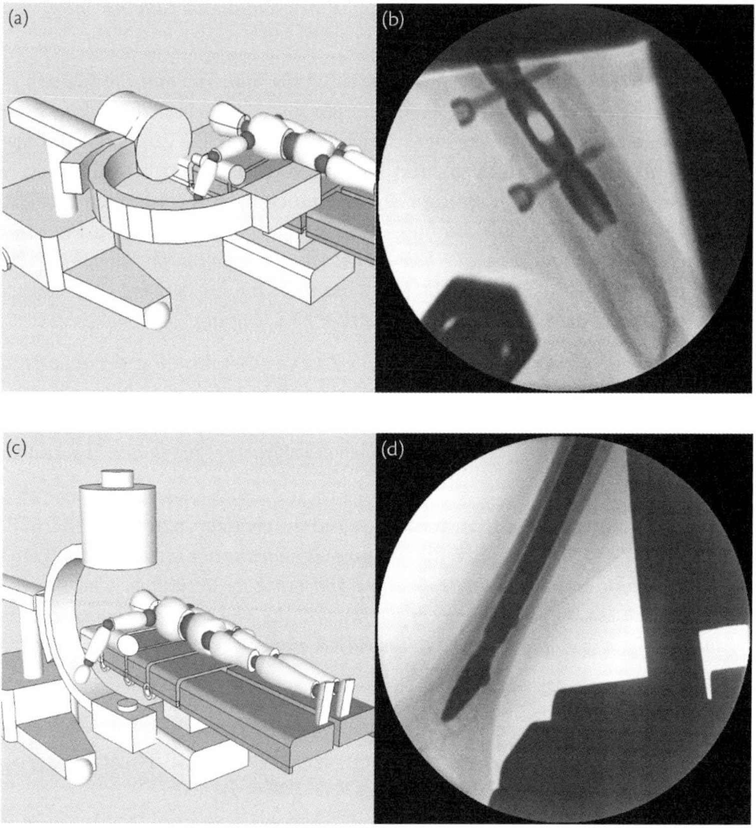

Figure 9.8 Prone position for retrograde humeral nail. (a) Lateral view of elbow in prone position. (b) Resulting image showing proximal locking screws. (c) Anteroposterior view of elbow in prone position. (d) Resulting image.

(b) and (d) Reproduced courtesy of Radiology Department, Leeds Teaching Hospitals NHS Trust, UK.

- *Before the proximal locking screws are inserted, the reduction and alignment at the fracture site may be rechecked under AP and lateral views to identify any adjustments that need to be made to positioning before continuing.*
- The proximal screws are inserted freehand through the posterior surface of the humerus. *The C-arm is positioned so that it is centred over the proximal locking screws in the AP position.* The arm may be manipulated so that the locking holes appear perfectly round on the image. *The position of the*

locking hole in relation to the soft tissues is then found under the AP view, and the surrounding area opened.

- *A drill is then positioned onto the surface of the humerus and the location of the tip checked in multiple AP views, so that it is directly over the locking hole.* Once the positioning is correct, the surgeon will drill a guide hole for the screw through the humerus and locking hole. The depth of the hole is then measured, and an appropriate-sized locking screw inserted into the guide hole and through the nail. *A lateral view may be performed to demonstrate the depth of the guide hole and screw in relation to the humerus.* The second screw is inserted in the same manner. *Images showing the proximal locking screws in two planes should be saved for archiving.*
- A compression device may be attached to the distal nail at the insertion point. *If used, imaging of the fracture site will be required to judge the position and state of the reduction as compression is applied. Once the compression appears satisfactory, AP and lateral views of the fracture site should be saved for archiving.*
- The positioning jig is then removed, and an end-cap placed on the nail. *AP and lateral views of the distal humerus showing the insertion point and distal locking screws should be obtained and saved for archiving. These views, along with the AP and laterals of the fracture site and proximal humerus with locking screws, should be saved to the PACS along with the dose information.*

References

Robinson, C., Teoh, K., Baker, A., and Bell, L. 'Fractures of the Lesser Tuberosity of the Humerus', *Journal of Bone and Joint Surgery*, 91/3 (2009), 512–20.

Fakler, J., Hogan, C., Heyde, C., and John, T. 'Current Concepts in the Treatment of Proximal Humeral Fractures', *Orthopaedics*, 31/1 (2008), 42–51.

10

Distal humerus and elbow

The elbow and distal humerus are complex regions of anatomy that allow extensive articulation of the forearm. They can often be injured through trauma. If functionality of the limb is to be maintained, it is essential that they heal correctly. The regions must also undergo opposing forces from the muscles that move the arm, and these can separate fractures, causing delay or failure to heal. As such, the elbow is a complex region to perform surgery on.

10.1 Distal humerus plating

For fractures of the distal humerus that may compromise the function of the elbow, plates can be implanted for internal fixation. Typically, two plates are inserted to aid stability at the fractures and support both columns of the distal humerus. If the articular surface of the elbow is compromised, a Chevron osteotomy of the olecranon may also be performed to allow access. If performed, the olecranon will require fixation (in the form of a tension band wiring, covered in section 10.2) once the humerus fixation has been completed.

Patient position

- Lateral decubitus position, with the affected arm on top and extended anteriorly to the patient; the elbow flexed over a radio-lucent support; and the forearm allowed to hang downwards
- Alternatively, prone with the affected limb abducted to 90° and supported on a radio-lucent support, and the elbow flexed downwards

C-arm approach

- From the head or foot end of the table and parallel with the patient's torso, with the C-arm centred over the posterior margin of the distal humerus of the affected limb

Key imaging

- *AP/lateral views of reduction*
- *AP/lateral views of fixation of condyles*
- *AP/lateral views of fit and size of plates*
- *AP/lateral views of screws*
- *AP/lateral/oblique/functional views of elbow for reduction and articulations*

Procedure

- The patient is positioned in either the prone or decubitus position. *AP and lateral views may be performed at the start of the case before cleaning and draping to identify any displaced fragments.* Manipulation of the joint under imaging can also help identify unstable fractures and potential problems with restoring articulation at the joints. Once this has been performed, the C-arm is withdrawn, and the region is cleaned and draped. The C-arm is also draped at this point (Figure 10.1).
- The region is opened, and, if required, the olecranon is cut in a V-shape (Chevron osteotomy) to allow access to the articular surface. The fracture site is cleared of clots and fragments. All the bone fragments involved are identified and located at this point. Loose areas of bone may be removed and the integrity of the articular surfaces checked.
- *If the fractures affect the articular surface of the distal humerus, this section will be reduced first.* The fracture segments are manipulated into anatomical position, and may be held with bone clamps while K-wires are inserted across the condyles. *The integrity of the surface and the position of the K-wires may be checked under imaging at this point in AP and lateral views.*
- Screws are then implanted either over or in place of the wires, and the wires removed.
- *The condyles are then reattached to the humerus.* The segments of the distal humerus are manually reduced to anatomical position before the segments are provisionally fixed with K-wires. The plates are then placed against the distal humerus to establish the size and fit. *Imaging may be required at this point to demonstrate the position of the plates against the bone and reduction of the fracture in AP and lateral views.* The plates are then removed and contoured to better fit the limb and rechecked until satisfactory.
- *If a posterior plate is being used, it is attached first.* The condyles are manipulated onto the distal end of the humerus, and a K-wire is driven

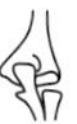

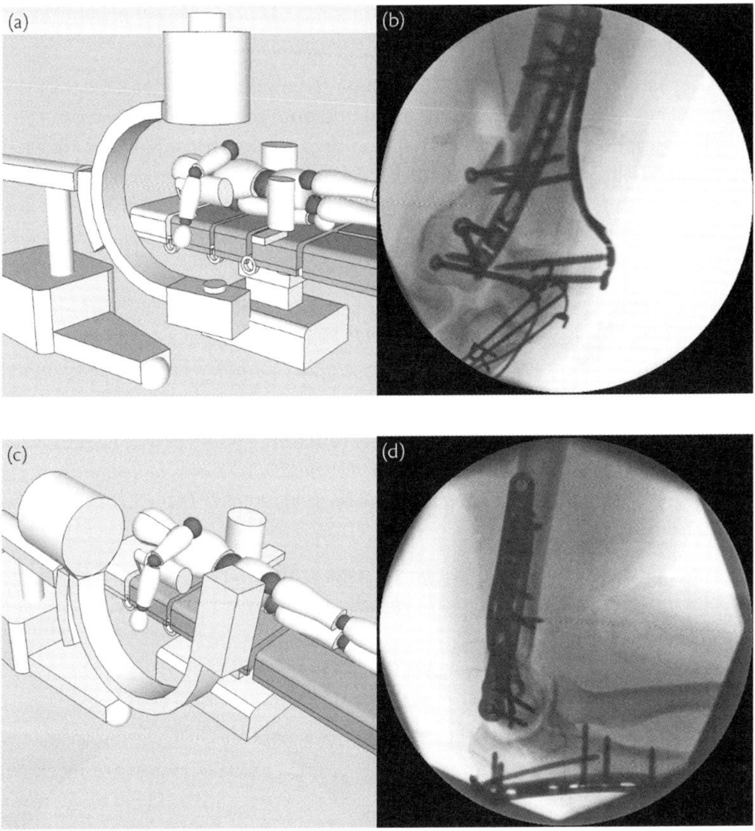

Figure 10.1 Decubitus position for elbow. (a) Anteroposterior view of distal humerus in decubitus position. Note body supports and arm support. (b) Resulting image (medial and posterior plates and olecranon wiring *in situ*). (c) Horizontal beam lateral view of distal humerus. (d) Resulting image.

(b) and (d) Reproduced courtesy of Radiology Department, Leeds Teaching Hospitals NHS Trust, UK.

through the distal end of the first plate into the condyles. The plate is then laid against the humerus and a proximal screw implanted to hold the plate against the limb. Further screws are then implanted through the plate to attach it to the limb and to support the fracture segments (Figure 10.2).

- The second plate is then attached with screws to the medial side of the limb. *Imaging in AP and lateral views will be required to check the position of the screws for the medial plate to ensure they do not strike the posterior plate screws and to check the integrity of the reduction.*

- Alternatively, plates can be attached on the medial and lateral sides of the humerus. The condyles are manipulated onto the distal humerus and the plates applied to each side so that they grip the condyles. K-wires are then inserted through the plates into the condyles and limb as a temporary fixation and as a guide for the screws. *Imaging may be required in AP and lateral views at this point to check the location of the wires within the limb and across the fracture sites.*
- The plates are then affixed to the condyles and humerus with screws replacing the K-wires. *Imaging in AP and lateral views may be required at this point to ensure that the screws do not collide within the limb or compromise the reduction.*
- Once the plates are fully attached, any remaining K-wires will be removed. *Images should be saved at this point in AP and lateral views to demonstrate the position of the plates and screws around the limb, as well as the reduction of the fractures.*
- If a Chevron osteotomy was performed at the start of the case, then the olecranon will now be fixed (typically via a tension band wiring of the olecranon).

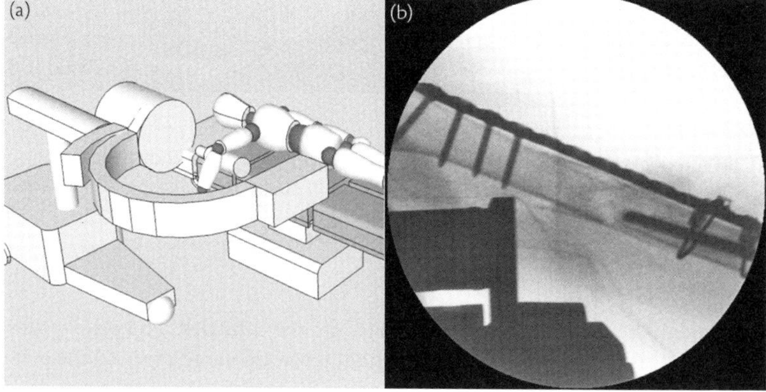

Figure 10.2 Prone/decubitus lateral humerus view. (a) Proximal lateral humerus approach. (b) Resulting image showing midshaft of humerus. Note: stem of elbow implant is visible.

(b) Reproduced courtesy of Radiology Department, Leeds Teaching Hospitals NHS Trust, UK.

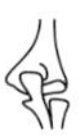

- *Once the fixation is completed and the clamps holding the incisions are removed, final AP and lateral views will be required to demonstrate the fixations and anatomy.* Oblique or functional views may also be required to demonstrate individual parts of the fixation and to ensure that the articulations of the limb are not compromised. *These images must be sent to the picture archiving and communication system (PACS) along with the dose summary.*

10.2 **Tension band wiring of olecranon**

Fractures across the articular surfaces of the olecranon are often displaced by the extensor muscles acting on the ulna. Because of this, it is often necessary to hold the fracture together in compression by tension wiring. Alternatively, the olecranon may have to be cut to access the articular surfaces of the elbow if there is an intra-articular fracture of the distal humerus (Chevron osteotomy). A tension band wiring is used to hold the fracture or osteotomy in anatomical reduction and ensure even forces across the fracture site. This prevents separation or deformity due to the muscles acting on the olecranon and ulna.

Patient position

- Lateral decubitus position, with the affected arm on top and extended anteriorly to the patient; the elbow flexed over a radio-lucent support; and the forearm allowed to hang downwards

C-arm approach

- From the head or foot end of the table and parallel with the patient's torso, with the C-arm centred over the posterior margin of the distal humerus of the affected limb

Key imaging

- *AP/lateral views for reduction of olecranon*
- *AP/lateral views for insertion of K-wires across fracture/osteotomy site*
- *AP/lateral views for reduction under tension*

Procedure

- The area is cleaned and the patient draped. *A sterile U-drape may also be wrapped around the base of the C-arm to prevent contamination by the X-ray tube.* As the surgeon also needs repeated access to this area during the procedure, it will be necessary to pull out the C-arm to allow access and then to recentre when imaging is required.

- The region posterior to the olecranon is opened, and the fracture site is located, cleaned, and manipulated into anatomical position. *It is then held in reduction with bone clamps, and the position checked in AP and lateral views* (Figure 10.3).
- A K-wire is inserted from the tip of the olecranon across the fracture/osteotomy site into the proximal ulna. *The position of this wire will be checked*

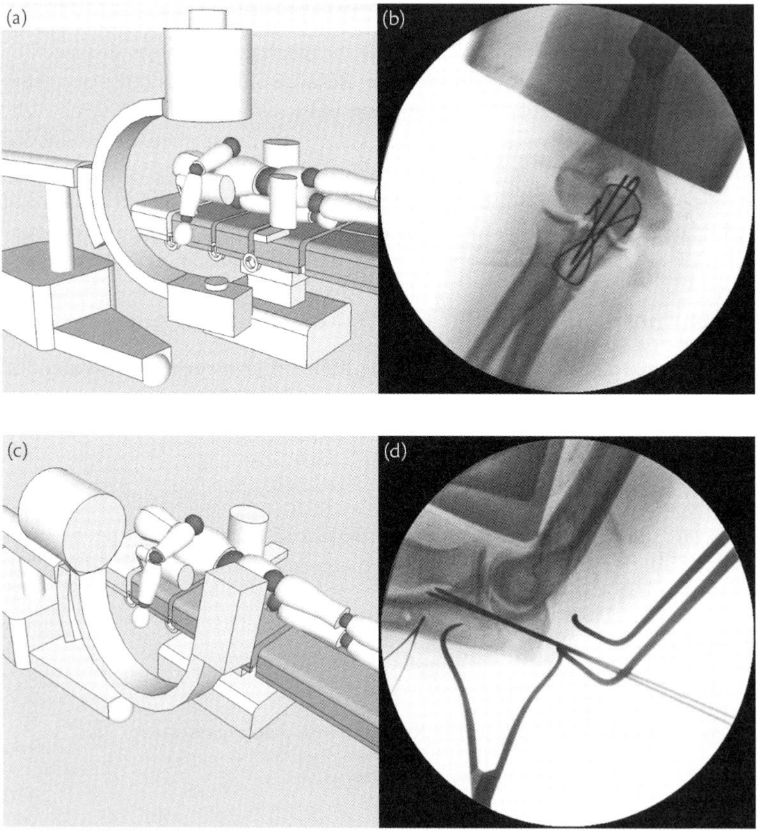

Figure 10.3 Decubitus position of elbow. (a) Anteroposterior (AP) positioning of distal humerus and elbow. (b) Resulting image, with tension band wiring in place. Forearm is raised, so that it is parallel to the floor to demonstrate olecranon in AP. (c) Horizontal beam lateral approach for lateral olecranon and distal humerus. (d) Resulting lateral image, with reduction clamp and guidewires visible.

(b) and (d) Reproduced courtesy of Radiology Department, Leeds Teaching Hospitals NHS Trust, UK.

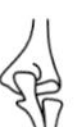

under AP and lateral views to ensure it is sufficiently within the bone and does not impinge on the articular surfaces. A second wire is then implanted parallel to and using the first as a guide.

- A hole is drilled across the proximal ulna, and a cable is threaded through it. This cable is then threaded in a figure of '8' pattern, with the loop over the ends of the K-wires and the crossover point on the posterior aspect of the ulna.
- The cable loop is tightened by twisting the ends together at the crossover point, pulling the fracture site into compression. *The reduction will be checked again in AP and lateral views under X-ray before the ends of the K-wires are bent round to form loops.*
- Once the reduction and fixation is deemed satisfactory, the ends of the K-wires are clipped and bent into loops so that the ends are against the olecranon. *Final AP and lateral views are taken, along with obliques to check the integrity of the joint surface if necessary. These images are sent to the PACS along with the dose summary.*

10.3 **Plate fixation of olecranon**

For more complex fractures of the olecranon, or where tension banding would not be practical (such as in osteoporotic bone), plates and screws can be used as a fixation.

Patient position

- Lateral decubitus position, with the affected arm on top and extended anteriorly to the patient; the elbow flexed over a radio-lucent support; and the forearm allowed to hang downwards

C-arm approach

- From the head or foot end of the table and parallel with the patient's torso, with the C-arm centred over the posterior margin of the distal humerus of the affected limb

Key imaging

- *AP/lateral views for reduction*
- *Lateral view for fit and sizing of plate*
- *AP/lateral views for insertion of lag screw (if used)*
- *AP/lateral/oblique views for insertion of screws*

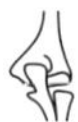

Procedure

- The area is cleaned and the patient draped. *A sterile U-drape may also be wrapped around the base of the C-arm to prevent contamination by the X-ray tube.* As the surgeon also needs repeated access to this area during the procedure, it will be necessary to pull out the C-arm to allow access and then to recentre when imaging is required.

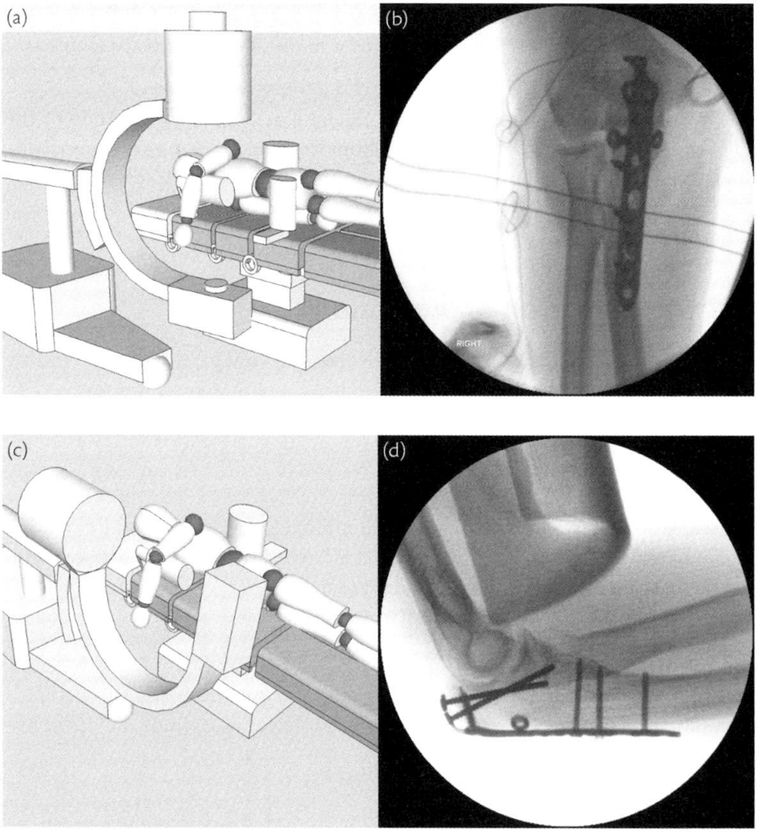

Figure 10.4 Decubitus positioning for olecranon plate. (a) Decubitus anteroposterior (AP) position of L elbow. Note body supports. (b) AP image, with olecranon plate *in situ*. (c) Decubitus lateral position of L elbow. (d) Resulting image. Note humerus support.

(b) and (d) Reproduced courtesy of Radiology Department, Leeds Teaching Hospitals NHS Trust, UK.

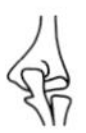

- The region posterior to the olecranon is opened, and the fracture site is located, cleaned, and manipulated into anatomical position. *It is then held in reduction with bone clamps, and the position checked in AP and lateral views.*
- A plate is selected and measured against the posterior surface of the olecranon and ulna. *A lateral view of the elbow may be required at this point to demonstrate the fit of the plate against the bone.* The plate may then be contoured for a better fit against the bone before it is implanted.
- In the case of an oblique fracture to the olecranon, a hole may be drilled across the fracture site for a lag screw. *The path of the drill will be checked in both AP and lateral views.* Once the position of the guide hole appears satisfactory, the depth will be measured, and a correctly sized lag screw is inserted into the guide hole and tightened to compress the fracture site. *A lateral view may be required to check the position of the fracture site and articular surfaces as compression is applied* (Figure 10.4).
- Further screws are then implanted through the proximal and distal regions of the plate to secure it to the bone. *Once these are implanted, their positions may be checked under AP and lateral views, and oblique views used to check for any screws around the articular surfaces.*
- *Once the reduction and fixation are satisfactory, final views in AP and lateral (plus any required obliques) are taken and archived in the PACS along with the dose information.*

11

Forearm and wrist

The wrist is one of the most commonly injured regions of the body, as it is used with the hands to protect the body and head when falling. The forearm is more often injured in direct trauma (such as a blow to the midshaft of the ulna), but any injuries to it may also affect the articulations at the wrist or elbow.

11.1 Radius and ulna

Due to the ring of bone formed by the radius and ulna, it is difficult to fracture one without an associated contrecoup injury. This may consist of a fracture or dislocation at the wrist or elbow, or a fracture to the shaft of both bones. The full method of how an open reduction internal fixation (ORIF) of the forearm is performed will vary if both the radius and ulna are involved, and according to the complexity and location of each fracture. A full guide to every possible procedure is unnecessary from the radiographer's perspective, and hence a plating of an isolated midshaft fracture will be covered here. If both the radius and ulna are fractured, one bone will undergo a preliminary fixation before the second bone is approached.

Patient position

- Supine, with the affected limb abducted at 90° and supported on a radiolucent table extension

C-arm approach

- At 90° to the affected limb, from either the head or foot end of the table, with the receptor centred over the radius and ulna

Key imaging

- *AP/lateral views for closed and open reductions*
- *AP/lateral views for fitting of plate*
- *AP/lateral views for insertion of lag screw*
- *AP/lateral views for insertion of screws to secure plate*

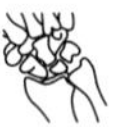

- *AP/lateral views of fracture site once compression is applied*
- *AP/lateral/functional views of plate, elbow, and wrist once fixation is completed*

Procedure

- *Closed reduction may take place under imaging control at the start of the case.* The integrity of the wrist and elbow joints may also be checked under live screening. *AP and lateral views are performed by the surgeon who is manipulating the arm on the table. However, if the reduction is unstable, some rotation of the C-arm may also be used to produce a second view with less manipulation of the limb in horizontal beam lateral (HBL) view.*
- The area around the fracture site is opened, and a preliminary reduction is performed. *Bone clamps may be used to hold the reduction in position and the fracture site checked under AP and lateral views.*
- A plate is applied to the bone. *This may require imaging in AP and lateral views to check the fit and contact of the plate against the bone.* This is especially required if the full length of the plate in place cannot be directly seen by the surgeons (e.g. the plate is inserted through a small incision).
- The plate may be removed and contoured to better fit against the bone, and may be bent into a slight curve, which will help compress the fracture site once attached.
- A lag screw may now be inserted in a guide hole across the fracture site to hold it in compression. *The direction of the drill bit is checked in relation to the fracture under AP and lateral imaging before drilling begins.* As the hole is drilled, more imaging may be required to check the drill path and integrity of the reduction. Once the guide hole is satisfactory, the depth is measured and an appropriate-sized screw is inserted (Figure 11.1).
- The plate is now attached to the bone. The first screw is attached through the plate via a guide hole in the same manner as the lag screw. The second screw is then inserted in the same manner, on the other side of the fracture site. *These two screws will induce compression at the fracture site, and, as such, imaging may be required again at the site to check the reduction.* Once the reduction appears satisfactory, more screws will be inserted into the plate in the same manner to secure it against the bone.
- *Once the final screws have been inserted, the fracture site and plate will be checked under imaging in AP and lateral views.* These images should be saved. *The wrist and elbow joints may also be checked for integrity under AP and lateral views, and may require some live screening to check for any irregularities in the functioning of the joints.* These images should also be saved. *Once the integrity of the limb is satisfactory, the C-arm can be withdrawn and all saved*

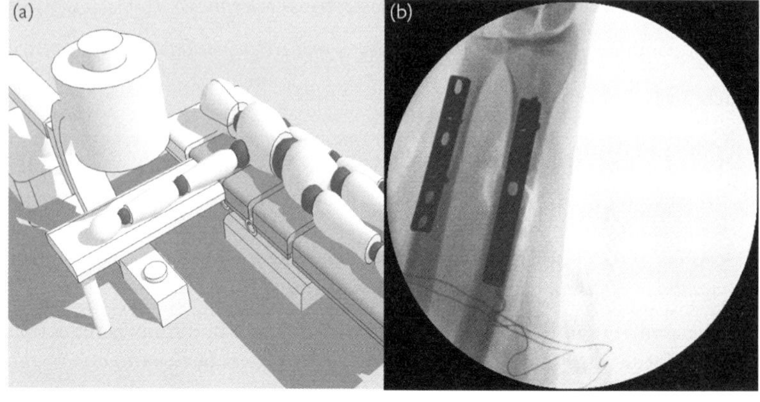

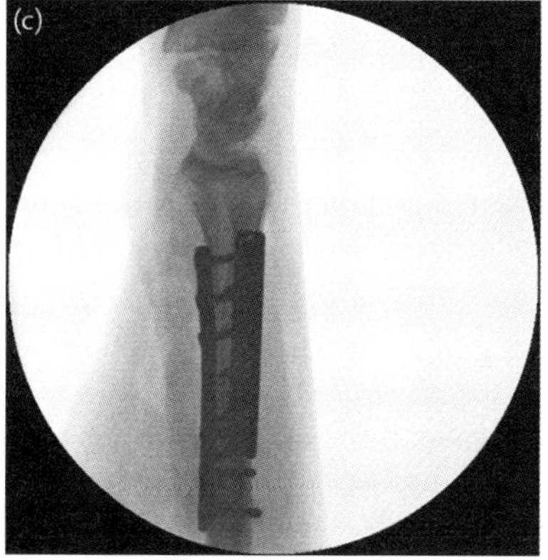

Figure 11.1 Supine position for radius and ulna. (a) Example of C-arm approach for right radius and ulna. (b) Anteroposterior image of radius and ulna demonstrating plates *in situ* on both bones. (c) Lateral view (performed by surgeon rotating the limb).
(b) and (c) Reproduced courtesy of Radiology Department, Leeds Teaching Hospitals NHS Trust, UK.

images archived to the picture archiving and communication system (PACS) along with the dose information.

11.2 **Wrist**

Wrists are one of the most common areas to be injured, often from falls onto an outstretched hand. Casting and closed manipulation will result in satisfactory outcomes in many wrist injuries. However, where the reduction of a

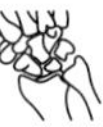

fracture cannot be maintained or the integrity of the wrist joint is affected, surgery may be required. The nature and stability of the fracture, quality of bone, and the patient's level of activity and hand dominance will all be taken into account before a decision to operate is made.

Patient position

- Supine, with the affected limb outstretched on a radio-lucent support

C-arm approach

- At around 90° to the patient's arm, from the side opposite/at 90° to the surgeon

Key imaging

- *AP/lateral views for closed reduction*
- *AP/lateral views for insertion of fixations*
- *AP/lateral views for checking of reduction*
- *AP/lateral/oblique/stress views for integrity of joint surface*

Procedure

- The wrist may be positioned with the palm facing up or down, depending on the region where the fixation is to be implanted, and on the surgeons' preference. *However, throughout the procedure, the arm will be moved between positions as the case progresses.*
- If possible, a closed reduction and fixation with K-wires is performed. *The fracture site is manually reduced with angulation of the distal segment removed. This will be checked under AP and lateral views.* Other views to check the integrity of the wrist joint (such as lateral-oblique) may also be required. These may be performed before the skin is cleaned and the patient and receptor are draped, and then rechecked after cleaning and draping. The C-arm should be withdrawn and draped over the receptor head once the reduction has been achieved and the skin is being cleaned (Figure 11.2).
- The skin is opened over the radial styloid process, and a K-wire is positioned with the tip onto the bone. *The angle of the wire is checked under AP view before the wire is driven into the bone and across the fracture site. The progress is checked under AP view before a lateral view is performed to check the position within the radius.*
- A second wire may also be inserted from the radial styloid process, so that it is nonparallel to the first. This will be inserted in the same manner.

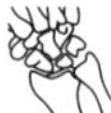

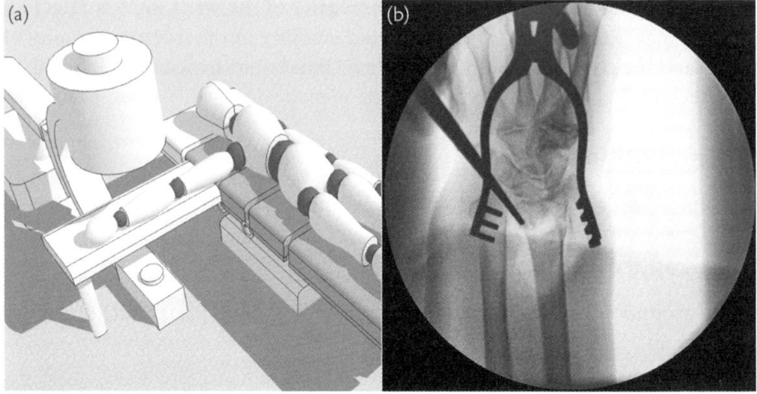

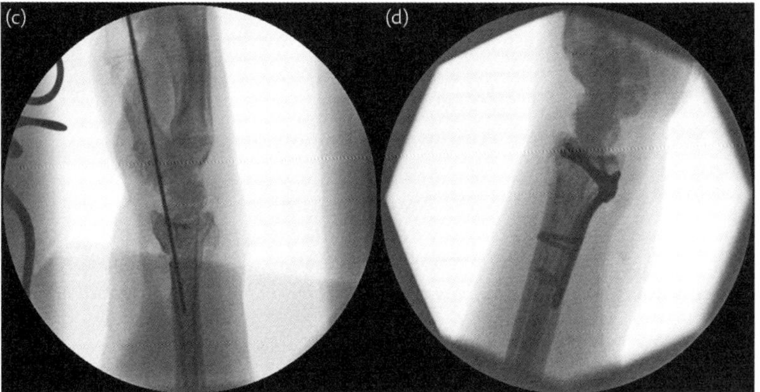

Figure 11.2 Supine position for wrist. (a) Approach for R wrist on table support. (b) Anteroposterior image with wrist opened. Note linear collimators, and density artefact from support below wrist joint. (c) Lateral image performed by rotating the arm. K-wire is being inserted. (d) Lateral image with wrist plate *in situ*.

(b), (c), and (d) Reproduced courtesy of Radiology Department, Leeds Teaching Hospitals NHS Trust, UK.

- A third wire can then be inserted from the medial dorsal region of the radius, so that it crosses over the first two wires. *This will be inserted in the same manner, with the position of the wire checked under imaging.*
- The wires are then cut to length and the protruding ends bent into hooks, to prevent them from migrating further into the bone and to aid removal. *Final images of the wrist are then taken, demonstrating the reduction and wire position, as well as the integrity of the wrist joint.*

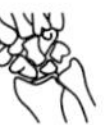

- *Alternatively, a plate may be inserted to support the reduction.* For injuries requiring ORIF to the distal ulna, the medial side of the wrist is opened and the fracture is manually reduced. *The position of the fracture and integrity of the articular surfaces are checked under AP and lateral views before the fixations are implanted.*
- The fracture may be fixed with a lag screw if applicable, which will be inserted across the fracture site under imaging control.
- A plate is then inserted along the shaft of the bone so that it extends beyond the fracture site in both directions. *The position and fit of the plate as well as the integrity of the fracture site are checked under AP and lateral views, as are the distal radio-ulnar joint and integrity of the wrist.*
- The plate is then attached to the bone with screws. Typically, the long section of the plate will be attached to the shaft of the radius first. *AP and lateral views may be required to check the position of the plate and screws, depending on the surgeon's preference.*
- *Distal screws are then implanted through the plate into the wrist.* These screws may be used to attach any comminuted fragments of the distal radius back onto the bone. The styloid process, in particular, can be reattached if avulsed in this manner. *AP and lateral views may be required to check the reduction and path of the screws.*
- *Once the reduction of the region appears satisfactory, the articulations of the wrist may be checked under X-ray.* This may consist of stress views with the wrist flexed from side to side, in dorsal flexion or palmar flexion, and oblique lateral views to show the distal radial surface in profile. Oblique views may also be performed to demonstrate the paths of the distal screws into the wrist and to check that they do not protrude into the articular surfaces. *Such views will depend on the positions of the screws and should be saved for archiving once acquired.*
- If there is any shortening of the radius due to the fracture, this will be corrected by extending the distal radius section of the plate until the alignment between the distal radius and ulna appears satisfactory. The long section of the plate will then be reattached to the shaft of the radius.
- Final images may then be taken with all temporary fixations and surgical aids removed. *This will consist of AP and lateral views, with the necessary stress or oblique views as well. These images should be transferred to the PACS along with the dose information.*

12

Pelvis

The pelvis is a complex area of anatomy, and fractures to it may be stable or unstable, depending on the location and nature of the injury. Lower-energy trauma may result in avulsion fractures and stable injuries that can be treated conservatively. High-energy trauma to the pelvis can result in unstable combinations of primary and contrecoup fractures, often associated with vascular, neurological, gynaecological, bladder, and rectal injuries, as well as trauma to other regions of the body, depending on the mechanism of injury. Such injuries are medical emergencies and will require surgical fixation. Typically, surgical fixation of pelvic fractures will take place in a major trauma centre, with a specialist surgical team performing the operation. Basic positioning and imaging technique for pelvic surgery will be covered here; however, the nature and location of the fracture will define the fixation used. Communication with the surgeons during such procedures is of paramount importance to ensure good demonstration of the required anatomy. If there are any uncertainties as to what is required, it is best to discuss these with the team as early as possible.

Procedure

- The patient is positioned supine on a radio-lucent table and should be moved so that the pelvis is as far down from the central column as possible. This will allow the C-arm to be angled over the relevant anatomy without the tube striking on the table.
- The C-arm is draped and brought in at 90° to the patient's midline, typically from the opposite side to the surgeon. However, it is possible that the surgical team will be working on both sides of the patient, so the C-arm may have to be withdrawn and repositioned when imaging is required (Figure 12.1).
- The region of the pelvis undergoing the procedure will be accessed. For structures on the inside of the pelvis, this will involve moving the overlying structures away from the region. This can take a significant amount of time.

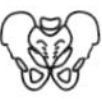

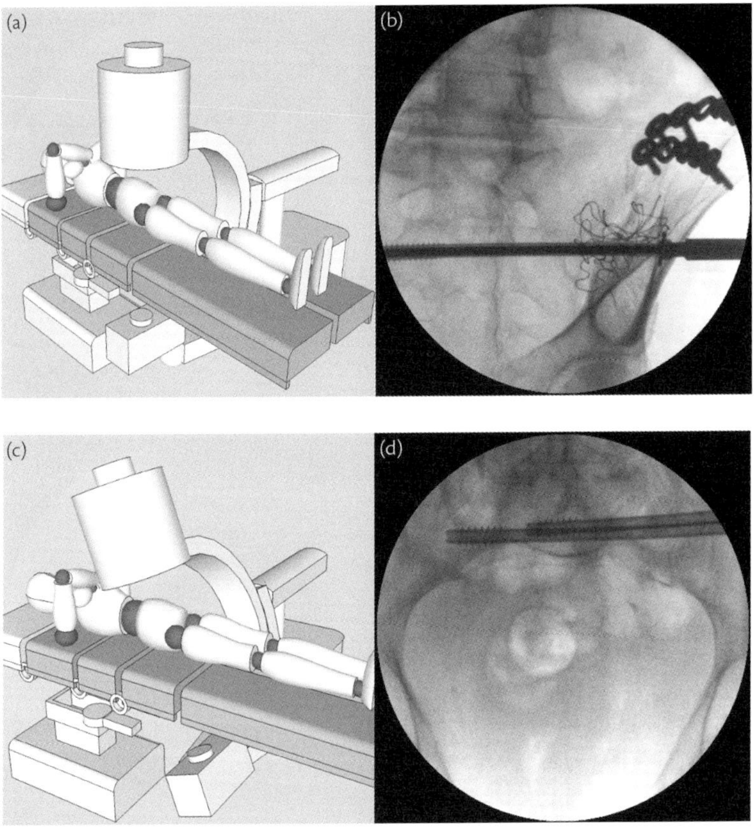

Figure 12.1 Pelvis imaging. (a) Anteroposterior view of pelvis approach from left side. (b) Resulting image, with SIJ screw inserted, iliac plates, swabs visible. (c) Outlet view position. (d) Resulting image, showing SIJ screws.

(b) and (d) Reproduced courtesy of Radiology Department, Leeds Teaching Hospitals NHS Trust, UK.

- Once the region is accessed, the reduction will take place. This will require imaging in at least two views, depending on the region (Figure 12.2).
- Once enough reduction is achieved to start fixation, imaging will be required to check the fit and path of any implants used. For plates used on the ilium, the fit and shape may have to be adjusted several times before it is satisfactory.

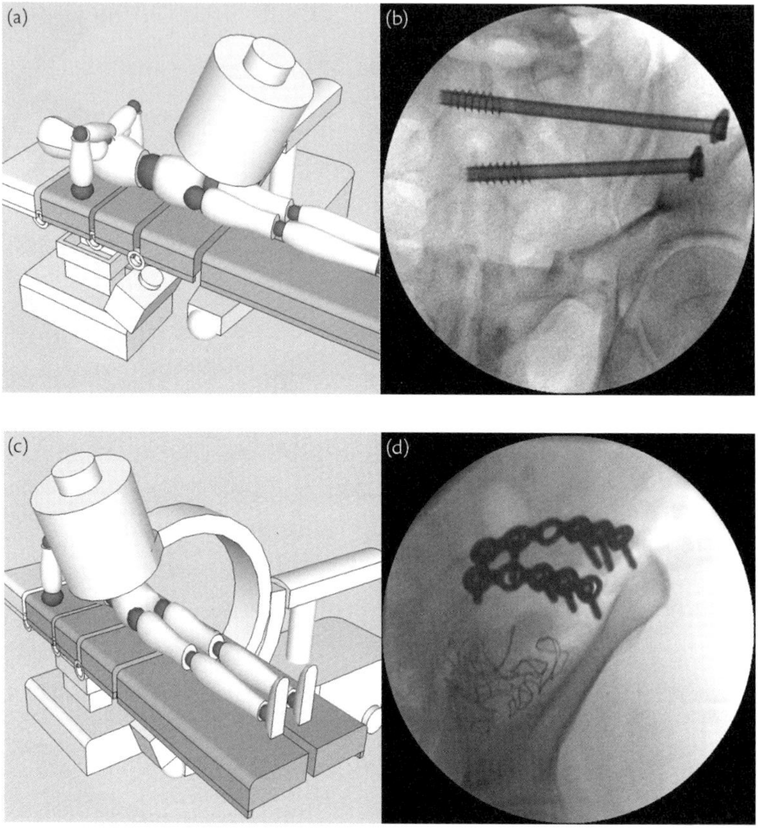

Figure 12.2 Further pelvis positioning. (a) Inlet view position. (b) Resulting image showing SIJ screws *in situ* (note rami fracture). (c) Right anterior oblique view centred over R iliac crest (can move to L crest to show face on). (d) Iliac crest end-on view, with plates and swabs visible.

(b) and (d) Reproduced courtesy of Radiology Department, Leeds Teaching Hospitals NHS Trust, UK.

- As the implant is attached to the bone, the reduction and path of the screws will be checked under imaging. Each separate region undergoing fixation will have to be checked individually as it is adjusted and fixation is applied (Figure 12.3).
- If screws are to be inserted into the sacroiliac joint, then an incision is made at the relevant side down to the bone. A guidewire is then drilled

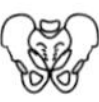

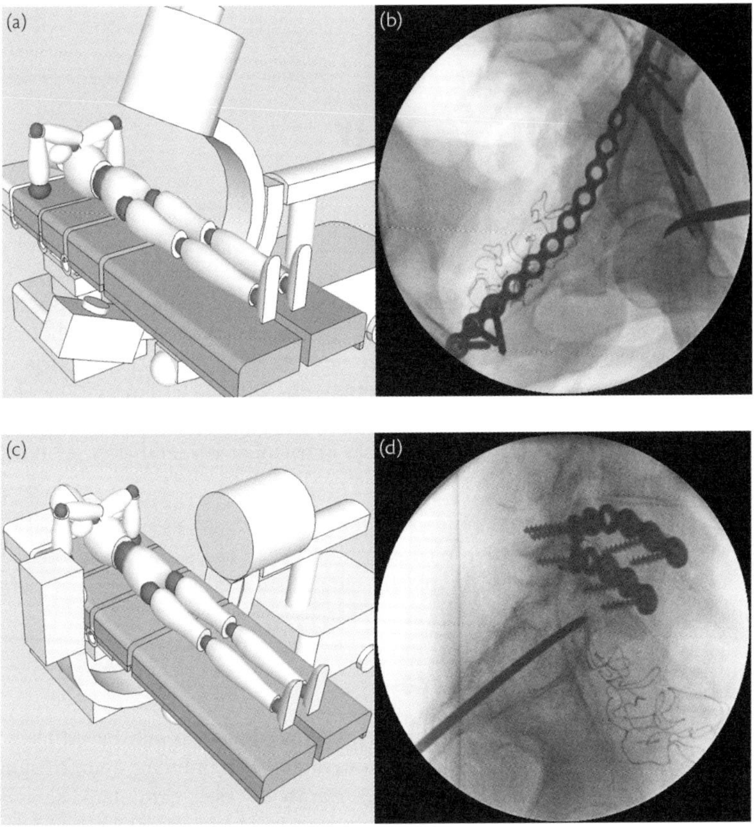

(a)

(b)

(c)

(d)

Figure 12.3 Additional pelvis imaging. (a) Left anterior oblique (LAO) view centred over L iliac crest (can move to R crest to show face on). (b) L acetabulum in LAO view showing plate and screws. (c) Lateral view approach. (d) Resulting image showing plates *in situ*.

(b) and (d) Reproduced courtesy of Radiology Department, Leeds Teaching Hospitals NHS Trust, UK.

through into the sacrum. Images in at least two views will be required to check the path of the guidewire before a screw is inserted either over the guidewire or into the guide hole.

- Once all fixation is implanted, final images in multiple views showing each fracture and all of the implants will be required. *These should be archived to the picture archiving and communication system along with the dose report.*

13

Hip and femur

Fractures of the hip are associated with various complications and delays in healing due to the patients' loss of mobility and independence. Patients with untreated or conservatively managed hip fractures may often be bed-bound and will require intensive nursing and care. As such, early intervention is currently seen as the optimal course for patients with such injuries. The rate of hip fractures is likely to continue to grow globally as people continue to live longer, leading to a rise in incidences of osteoporosis (and associated insufficiency fractures).

The femur is the strongest bone in the human body, and, as such, injuries to it are often the result of high-energy trauma. Such cases may be associated with other injuries, and will typically require surgical intervention to help the limb heal.

13.1 Cannulated hip screw

For stable undisplaced fractures along the femoral neck, it may be sufficient to prevent any displacement or distraction rather than inducing compression (as with a dynamic hip screw, or DHS). For these cases, cannulated screws may be inserted into the hip. This procedure involves far smaller incisions than a DHS or total hip replacement (THR), but will require repeated imaging to assess the position of the implants within the femoral neck.

Patient position

- Supine on traction table, with contralateral leg flexed and abducted

C-arm approach

- Between the patient's legs, at 90° to the affected femoral neck, centred over the affected hip

Key imaging

- *AP/lateral views for reduction of fracture*

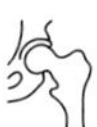

- *AP/lateral views for insertion of guidewires*
- *AP/lateral views for drilling over guidewire and insertion of screws*

Procedure

- *The patient is positioned supine onto a fracture table, with the affected limb close to the edge.* A perineal post is attached to the table between the patient's legs, and his or her feet are secured to the traction arms before the leg rests are removed. The unaffected limb is flexed at the hip and knee, and rotated outwards.
- *The C-arm is brought in at approximately 90° to the femoral neck, so that it can rotate underneath for a horizontal beam lateral (HBL) view without hitting the table or the patient.* Enough space should be given over the anterior aspect of the patient to allow rotation to the lateral view without adjusting the height of the centre column. For the lateral view, the C-arm is rotated under the patient, so that the receptor head is between the patient's legs. Be careful not to catch the receptor on the patient's leg, especially with larger patients. *If the femoral head/acetabulum is not sufficiently demonstrated on the lateral view, the centre column can be angled towards the patient, the receptor pushed closer to the hip, or the position of the base unit adjusted* (Figure 13.1).
- *The fracture is manipulated using the traction arm and the position checked under AP and lateral views.* This is a good time to see if anything is going to impinge on rotating the C-arm, as any adjustments can be more easily made now than once the patient is draped. Once reduction has been achieved, the C-arm is pulled out to allow cleaning and draping of the area.
- *The site is cleaned and draped. A sterile sheet is attached to the affected limb and hung from an overhead rail.* Once a lateral view is performed, the tube will carry up the drape with it as it rotates, keeping the tube covered, and the sterile side uncontaminated. While the C-arm is away from the patient as draping is taking place, it is often a good idea to wrap a nonsterile plastic bag over the X-ray tube, securing it with tape if necessary. This will protect the tube from blood spillage during the procedure, and will make cleaning the machine at the end of the case much easier.
- *A guidewire is mounted onto a drill and positioned at the hip. The angle and position of the wire in relation to the femoral neck will be checked under an AP view.* This may occur before any incision is made, so as to gauge the correct point from where to insert the wire. Alternatively, the incision may be made and the wire inserted through an aiming device.

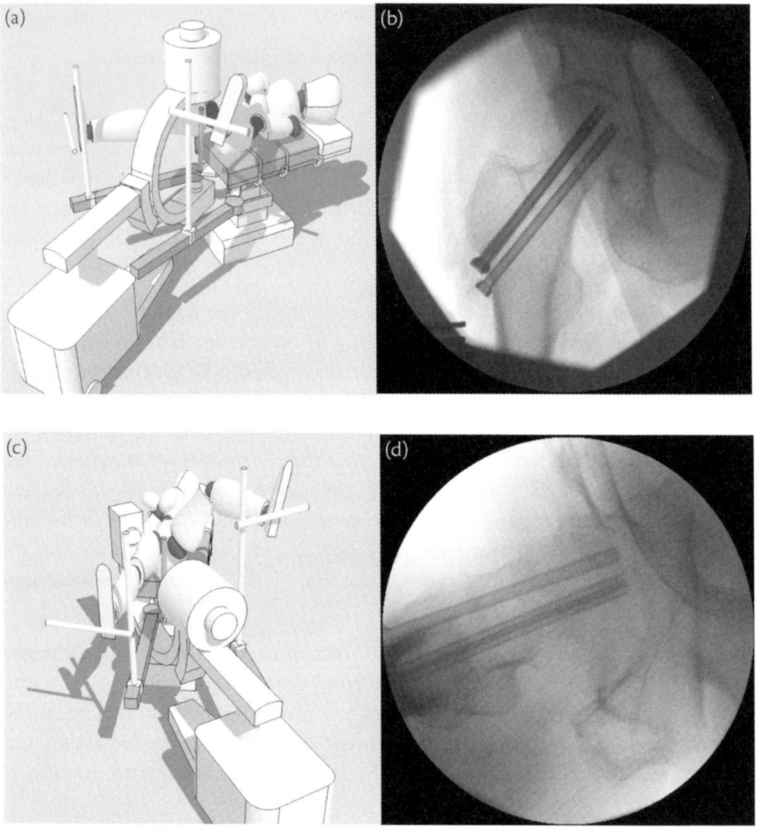

Figure 13.1 Cannulated hip screw position. (a) Anteroposterior (AP) position for R Hip, with left leg positioned to allow C-arm access. (b) AP image with hip screws *in situ*. Note: femoral head is not crossed by any screws. (c) Lateral position for R hip. (d) Lateral image with hip screws *in situ*.

(b) and (d) Reproduced courtesy of Radiology Department, Leeds Teaching Hospitals NHS Trust, UK.

- *The wire is advanced into the bone.* The depth and path of the wire will be checked using AP views, and with a lateral view once the depth appears satisfactory. If the wire is not in the correct location under both views, it may have to be withdrawn and reinserted.
- A second wire is then inserted parallel to the first. *The path and depth of this wire will also need to be checked under AP and lateral views as it is*

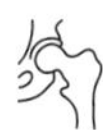

advanced. Once the wire appears in a satisfactory position, a third wire may also be inserted if needed.

- The length of the wires inside the hip are measured and screws selected to fit over the guidewires.
- *Guide holes are drilled over the wires using a cannulated drill.* The path of the drill and position of the fracture site are checked under imaging as the drill is advanced into the hip.
- *Cannulated screws are advanced over the wires into the hip.* The fit of the screws should be checked under AP view once they are inserted, to ensure the screw heads are against the lateral border of the hip.
- Once the position of the screws is satisfactory, the guidewires are removed. Final AP and lateral views of the hip with the screws in place and guidewires removed should then be taken. *These images should be transferred to the picture archiving and communication system (PACS) along with the dose information.*

13.2 Dynamic hip screw

The implantation of a sliding or dynamic hip screw (DHS) is one of the most commonly performed orthopaedic procedures. It consists of a broad threaded cancellous screw in the femoral head, which is then connected to a plate on the lateral aspect of the femur. This screw slides onto the femoral plate and allows movement between the two components, and hence it is 'dynamic'. The screw can either be left to slide freely (so that the patient's weight-bearing achieves compression at the fracture site), or a separate compression screw can be inserted at the end of the case that pulls the hip screw and plate together.

Patient position

- Supine on the traction table, with contralateral leg flexed and abducted

C-arm approach

- Between the patient's legs, at 90° to the affected femoral neck, centred over the affected hip

Key imaging

- *AP/lateral views for reduction of fracture*
- *AP/lateral views for insertion of guidewire*

- *AP/lateral views for drilling over guidewire and insertion of hip screw*
- *AP view for fitting of hip plate*

Procedure

- *The patient is positioned supine onto a fracture table, with the affected limb close to the edge.* A perineal post is attached to the table between the patient's legs, and his or her feet are secured to the traction arms before the leg rests are removed. The unaffected limb is flexed at the hip and knee, and rotated outwards.
- *The C-arm is brought in at approximately 90° to the femoral neck, so that it can rotate underneath for an HBL view without hitting the table or the patient.* Enough space should be given over the anterior aspect of the patient to allow rotation to the lateral view without adjusting the height of the centre column. For the lateral view, the C-arm is rotated under the patient so that the receptor head is between the patient's legs. Be careful not to catch the receptor on the patient's leg, especially with larger patients. *If the femoral head/acetabulum is not sufficiently demonstrated on the lateral view, the centre column can be angled towards the patient, the receptor pushed closer to the hip, or the position of the base unit adjusted* (Figure 13.2).
- *The fracture is manipulated using the traction arm, and the position checked under AP and lateral views.* This is a good time to see if anything is going to impinge on rotating the C-arm, as any adjustments can be more easily made now than once the patient is draped. Once reduction has been achieved, the C-arm is pulled out to allow cleaning and draping of the area.
- *The site is cleaned and draped. A sterile sheet is attached to the affected limb and hung from an overhead rail.* Once a lateral view is performed, the tube will carry up the drape with it as it rotates round, keeping the tube covered and the sterile side uncontaminated. While the C-arm is away from the patient as draping is taking place, it is often a good idea to wrap a nonsterile plastic bag over the X-ray tube, securing it with tape if necessary. This will protect the tube from blood spillage during the procedure, and make cleaning the machine at the end of the case much easier.
- *The soft tissues lateral to the hip are opened to allow access. A guidewire is mounted through an aiming device from below the greater trochanter up the middle of the femoral neck towards the head.* The position of the aiming device and wire in relation to the femoral neck will be checked via AP views before the wire is driven into the hip.

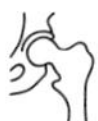

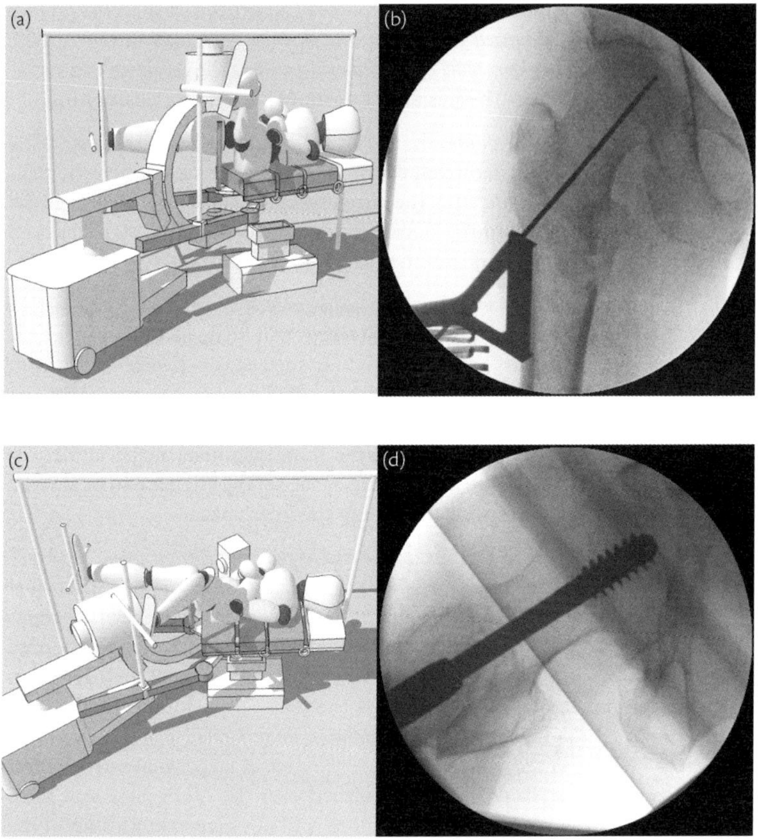

Figure 13.2 Dynamic hip screw (DHS) positioning. (a) Anteroposterior (AP) position for R hip. Note the frame used for hanging sterile drape (omitted here). (b) AP image with guidewire inserted through aiming device into femoral neck. (c) Lateral position for R hip. Sterile drape will be brought up on X-ray tube. (d) Lateral image showing DHS *in situ*. Note artefact from perineal post. This can be used to orientate the image.

(b) and (d) Reproduced courtesy of Radiology Department, Leeds Teaching Hospitals NHS Trust, UK.

- *The guidewire is driven through the aiming device through the femoral neck and fracture site.* The position is checked in AP view to ensure it is proceeding along the middle of the femoral neck and not penetrating into the joint space. If any implant diverges too far from the midline, it can cause unrecognized joint impingement even while appearing to be fully within

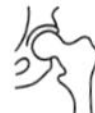

the femoral head on AP and lateral views (Noordeen et al. 1993). *Once the wire has been advanced far enough, the position is checked in lateral view to ensure it is within the middle of the femoral neck.* Oblique views can occasionally be used where there is any uncertainty regarding positioning.

- *In some cases, a second guidewire will be inserted, parallel to the first.* This prevents the femoral head from rotating out of alignment when the drill crosses the fracture site into the proximal segment. This wire will be inserted without the aiming device, with its position and path checked under imaging in the same manner as the first wire.
- *A cannulated drill is driven over the central guidewire, to create a channel for the hip screw.* As with the guidewire, images will be needed to ensure that the drill does not cross into the articular surface, or diverge away from the midline of the femoral neck. Once the drill position is satisfactory on the AP view, the lateral may be checked again. The drill is then removed, leaving the guidewire in place, and the screw segment of the implant is inserted over it. Again, the positioning of the screw will need to be viewed by X-ray to check for impingement into the joint space.
- *The compression plate is attached to the end of the compression screw, and cortical screws are used to attach it securely to the shaft of the femur.* Some surgeons may want AP screening of the plate to check whether the depth gauge is in place after drilling, and to confirm the length and positioning of the screws. If a compression screw is to be used, it will be inserted at this point and tightened to compress the femoral neck onto the body of the femur. *As this will affect the fracture site, imaging will be needed to ensure that the integrity of the reduction has not changed.* A larger plate (trochanter stabilization plate, or TSP) can be placed over the DHS plate and fixed with screws or wires where a DHS alone will not give enough stability to the hip.
- *The guidewire is removed, and the surrounding tissues are closed.* Final images can be captured, consisting of AP and lateral views of the femoral neck and plate. *These images should be transferred to the PACS along with the dose information.*

13.3 Antegrade femoral nailing

This implant consists of a long metal rod with holes for locking the screws at each end, and is inserted down the medullary canal of the femur. This implant offers very good support and fixation as well as allowing the patient to weight-bear on the limb earlier, although it may not be feasible where the canal is occluded by a pre-existing hip implant or other obstruction.

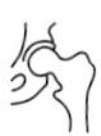

However, it is a widely performed procedure for femoral fractures, and can often be a challenge for radiographers who are unfamiliar with it.

Patient position

- Supine, with the contralateral leg flexed and abducted
- For distal locking, the contralateral leg is straightened and lowered below the affected leg

C-arm approach

- Between the patient's legs, at 90° to the affected femoral neck, centred over the affected hip
- For distal locking, centred over the knee at 90° to the femur from the contralateral side

Key imaging

- *AP/lateral views for the reduction of fracture*
- *AP/lateral views for the opening of insertion point*
- *AP view of full length of femur for the insertion of guidewire*
- *AP/lateral views for crossing fracture site with guidewire*
- *AP view of hip for measuring the length of the inserted guidewire*
- *AP view of full length of femur for the insertion of nail over guidewire*
- *AP/lateral views for the insertion of proximal locking*
- *Lateral/AP views of distal femur for the insertion of distal locking*

Procedure

- *The patient is positioned supine onto a fracture table, with the affected limb close to the edge.* A perineal post is attached to the table between the patient's legs, and his or her feet are secured to the traction arms before the leg rests are removed. The unaffected limb is flexed at the hip and knee, and rotated outwards.
- *The C-arm is brought in at approximately 90° to the femoral neck, so that it can rotate underneath for an HBL view without hitting the table or the patient.* Enough space should be given over the anterior aspect of the patient to allow rotation to the lateral view without adjusting the height of the centre column. For the lateral view, the C-arm is rotated under the patient so that the receptor head is between the patient's legs. Be careful not to catch

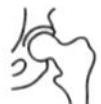

the receptor on the patient's leg, especially with larger patients. *If the femoral head/acetabulum is not sufficiently demonstrated on the lateral view, the centre column can be angled towards the patient, the receptor pushed closer to the hip, or the position of the base unit adjusted* (Figure 13.3).

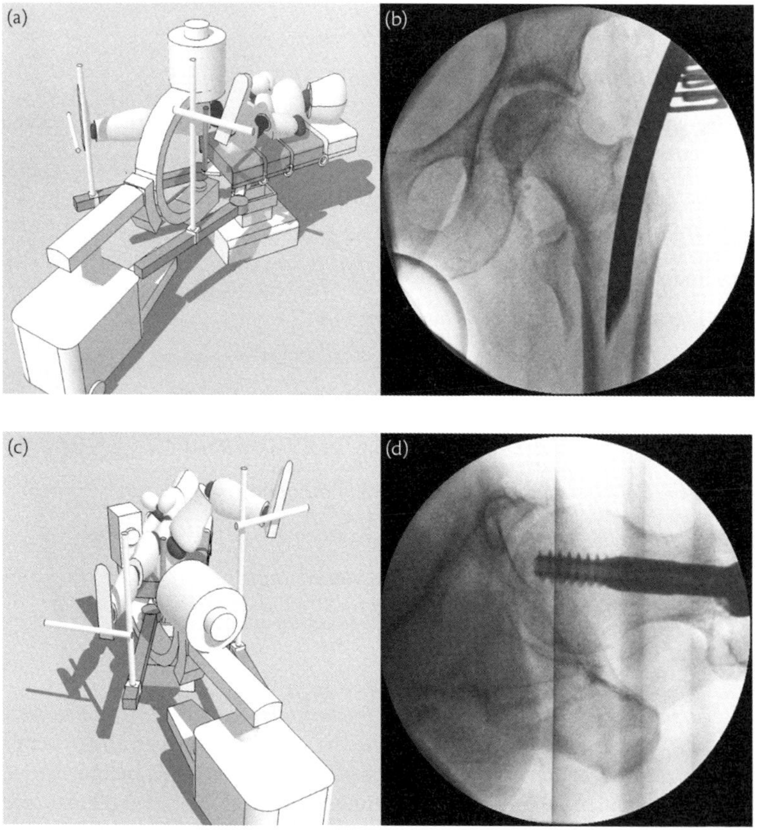

Figure 13.3 Antegrade femoral nailing. (a) Anteroposterior (AP) approach for R hip/proximal femur. Note abduction of L leg for C-arm access. (b) AP image showing widening of nail insertion point. Note avulsed lesser trochanter. (c) Lateral approach for R hip/proximal femur. (d) Resulting image.

(b) and (d) Reproduced courtesy of Radiology Department, Leeds Teaching Hospitals NHS Trust, UK.

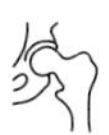

- *During the procedure, the C-arm will need to be repeatedly moved from the hip to the distal femur and back.* There must be no impediments for the C-arm along the length of the femur.
- For the lateral view, the C-arm is swung under the affected leg to horizontal beam, although the HBL of the femoral shaft will be more oblique when aligned for the femoral neck. For the majority of the case, this will suffice; however, for the implantation of the distal locking screws, a true anatomical lateral view is needed.
- *The fracture site is located in AP view before cleaning and draping of the patient takes place.* The surgeon will attempt to reduce the fracture by manipulating the limb via the traction arm at this point, with imaging used to check the position and alignment of the fracture site.
- If closed manipulation via the traction arm proves unsuccessful, the middle of the thigh may be supported from underneath with a brace. *If a support is used, it is important that this be far enough from the fracture site to allow the C-arm to image the fracture.* It is also important for the radiographer to remember that the support is in place, and to be careful to not strike it when moving the C-arm along the femur!
- When checking the alignment of the femur, the views of the hip should include the entire femoral neck and hip joint, as well as both trochanters. This allows the rotation of the leg to be judged correctly, and to avoid malrotation at the fracture site. Similarly, the fracture site will be checked for alignment and rotation. If the fracture is not multi-fragment, then there should not be a large difference between the width of the femur and intra-medullary (IM) canals between the proximal and distal parts of the fracture. Any discrepancy may indicate that the distal segment is out of rotational alignment with the proximal femur. Alternatively, an alignment guide may be laid over the femur, over the femoral head and down through the middle of the patella, and down to the ankle if needed. *The alignment can then be checked on X-ray against the guide* (Figure 13.4).
- *Once the AP view is satisfactory, alignment of the fracture site will be checked in the lateral view.* If reduction still cannot be achieved or maintained, the region of the fracture site can be opened, and surgical clamps or banding wires can be used to hold the femur in alignment.
- *Once closed reduction via manipulation has been successful (or abandoned in favour of open reduction), the C-arm is withdrawn to allow cleaning and draping of the patient.* If a hanging drape is used as in a DHS, the C-arm will not need to be draped. Otherwise, a sterile drape will need to be

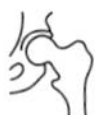

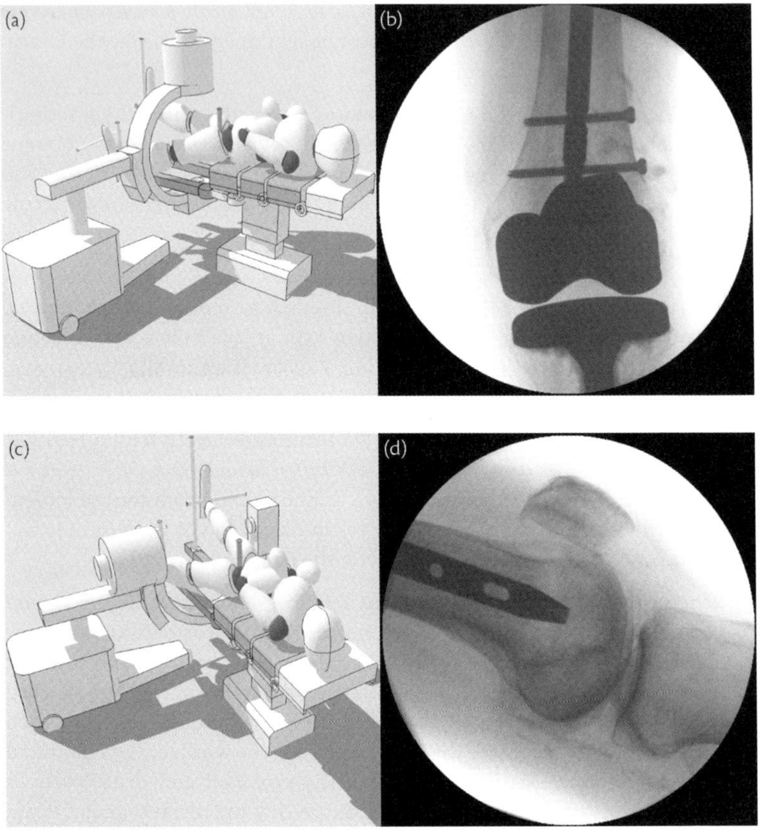

(a) (b) (c) (d)

Figure 13.4 Femoral nailing, distal position. (a) Anteroposterior (AP) view of R knee/distal femur. Note L leg is now lowered to allow for horizontal beam lateral (HBL) view of the knee. (b) Resulting AP image showing locking screws *in situ,* and total knee replacement. (c) HBL of R knee/distal femur. (d) Resulting image showing distal locking holes.

(b) and (d) Reproduced courtesy of Radiology Department, Leeds Teaching Hospitals NHS Trust, UK.

placed over the receptor head before the C-arm is brought back in and imaging can continue.

- *While the C-arm is away from the patient as draping is taking place, it is often a good idea to wrap a nonsterile plastic bag over the X-ray tube, securing it with tape if necessary.* This will protect the tube from blood spillage during the

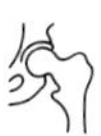

procedure, and will make cleaning the machine at the end of the case much easier.

- *The implant is inserted either through or medially to the greater trochanter.* Once the reduction of the fracture site is satisfactory, the entry point is located and checked under AP view. *The entry point should line up with the femoral canal, and so it is necessary to include a portion of the proximal femur on the AP image.*
- A short guidewire is inserted through the tissues to the desired entry point within the bony anatomy, and the position checked in AP view. Once the entry point appears satisfactory, a lateral view of the hip is required to check the anterior/posterior alignment. The entry point is then widened to allow access to the medullary canal via a cannulated drill over the wire. This may be performed under X-ray, especially if there is any risk of misalignment or loss of fracture reduction (e.g. in proximal femur fractures).
- *The nail itself is usually implanted over a guidewire, which is inserted down the length of the femur.* The wire is advanced down the femoral shaft, and the C-arm should track it in AP view to the fracture site.
- *The surgeon then crosses the fracture site with the wire, keeping it within the medullary canal of the distal femur.* AP views will be required, followed by a lateral view once the AP appears to demonstrate the wire in the distal segment. An angled lateral of the femur (i.e. with the beam horizontal but superior–inferior as with the lateral hip view) will suffice as opposed to a full 90° lateral view, as this will demonstrate if the nail is within the medullary canal.
- *For non-cannulated nails, which are not inserted over a wire, the nail is inserted once the entry point is opened.* Reaming is not performed. For these nails, X-ray is used to check the position as the nail is inserted down the femur, with lateral views at the fracture site to ensure it crosses into the distal segment correctly. However, these nails are far less commonly used than the cannulated nails covered here.
- *Once the guidewire is demonstrated in the distal femur, it is advanced again to just above the knee* (again, checked by AP view), where it will remain in place for the majority of the procedure. *It is often worth saving an AP of the distal femur (ideally with the articular surface of the knee included) to demonstrate the position of the guidewire in relation to the knee joint.*
- *Once the guidewire is in a good position, the size of the nail to be implanted can be decided.* The length of the nail can be assessed by either measuring off the guidewire (length of the wire – length of the unused portion over the

point of proximal locking = nail length), or by using a radio-lucent ruler over the femur.

- *For measuring off the wire, an AP view of the hip to demonstrate the proximal locking point may be required.* For the ruler technique, two AP views—an AP of the knee to align the end of the ruler with the tip of the wire, and then an AP of the hip—will be required to measure the distance to the proximal locking site. *When this is performed, the C-arm receptor must be parallel to the femur and the ruler, to prevent over/underestimation of the length of the femur.* Some surgeons may also decide on the nail width at this point, by checking the width of the femoral canal against the ruler. This is performed at the midshaft of the femur that represents the narrowest section of the IM canal.
- *Cannulated reamers are then introduced over the guidewire to widen the IM canal, starting with the narrowest gauge and gradually moving up in size.* Assuming that the guidewire is correctly in place, the reamers will progress straight down the middle of the IM canal and across the fracture site to the end of the wire. *However, in more unstable or difficult reductions, the surgeon may ask for imaging around the fracture site to ensure that the reamer does not veer off course or affect the alignment.*
- *Once reaming is completed, the nail is inserted over the wire. Imaging will be required in AP view to demonstrate that it is in place and has been advanced far enough within the femur.* As with the reamers, the process of crossing the fracture site with the nail can affect the reduction, and hence X-rays may be required. An AP demonstrating the end of the nail in relation to the knee may also be requested. *The guidewire is removed once the nail is in a satisfactory position.*
- *Once the nail is in position, it is locked by screws at the distal and proximal ends.* This prevents rotation and shortening at the fracture site, and locks the nail in place within the femur. The proximal locking screws are inserted either at the base of or into the femoral neck (hip screw), while the distal screws are inserted just above the epicondyles of the knee.
- The proximal locking screws may be implanted via a guide arm connected to the proximal segment of the nail itself. This system gives alignment for drilling and screw implantation through the proximal locking hole/s, depending on the surgical requirements. *If a hip screw is to be implanted into the femoral neck for proximal support, a semi-radio-lucent guide can be used to demonstrate the path and depth of the screw.* This connects to the drill guide and can swing around the hip and align with the locking holes in the nail in both AP and lateral views. *The path of the drill and the implantation of the*

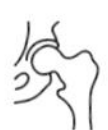

screw will also need to be checked on X-ray in the same manner as in a DHS, to ensure good bone contact and avoid joint impingement.

- Alternatively, screws can be inserted through the nail, locking it to the proximal femur rather than the hip. *AP and lateral views will be required to demonstrate them in place once they are inserted via the guide rig.* These images should be saved for archiving.
- The C-arm is now withdrawn, and the patient's unaffected leg is straightened and lowered so that it is beneath the affected limb.
- The distal locking screws are typically inserted under image guidance. To demonstrate the locking holes correctly, the beam must be aligned directly through them, so that both sides of the holes are perfectly overlaid without distortion. The C-arm is then brought in at 90° to the affected femur and rotated under the legs to HBL at the level of the distal femur.
- *A lateral view is now taken and adjustments made to the positions of both the C-arm and the leg in order to have the locking holes perfectly aligned on the image.* It is important to have the holes positioned as close to the centre of the receptor head as possible, as beam divergence will make true lateral alignment very difficult otherwise. *If the locking holes are not perfectly round in relation to the length of the nail, angling of the centre column can be used to improve alignment. If they are not perfectly circular perpendicular to the length of the nail, a slight rotation of the C-arm or rotation of the patient's leg via the traction arm can correct this.* Electronic magnification can help demonstrate the holes and identify any misalignment. Collimation to the region around the locking holes (with both the linear and iris diaphragms) can greatly improve the image quality and reduce the backscatter dose to the surgeon while performing this view. A sterile wire grid can be placed on the lateral side of the limb, above the condyles, to be used as a guide during imaging for where the locking holes are (Salvi 2008).
- *Once the C-arm and the nail are exactly aligned, the surgeon will open the skin over the locking holes and align the drill to them.* Multiple images will be used to check that the point of the drill is directly over the locking holes, and *the C-arm and leg must remain entirely still during this process.*
- *A screw hole is drilled through the distal femur and the nail holes by aligning the drill along the central ray.* The first locking screw is inserted. The procedure is then repeated for the second screw, often using the first as a guide for alignment.
- *The lateral and AP views of the distal screws should be saved*, and it is a good idea to open the collimation to demonstrate the distal end of the nail in

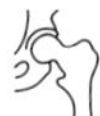

relation to the articular surface of the knee. At least one view of the fracture site (demonstrating the nail crossing it) should be saved, as well as an AP and lateral view of the proximal nail and hip. *These images should be saved and archived to the PACS along with the dose information.*

13.4 Retrograde femoral nailing

For fractures of the distal femur where the locking screws of an antegrade IM nail would be too close to the fracture site, a retrograde nail can be implanted. This can be either a much shorter nail, or a full-length nail that has proximal locking around the hip joint (as with an antegrade nail). Both types are introduced into the IM canal from the knee and advanced up the femur.

Patient position

- Supine, with the affected limb raised and flexed at the knee and the contralateral limb lowered, pelvis below centre column of table

C-arm approach

- From the contralateral side at 90° to the affected femur, centred over the knee, angled parallel to the femoral shaft

Key imaging

- *AP/lateral views of fracture site for closed reduction*
- *AP view of full length of femur*
- *AP/lateral views of knee*
- *AP oblique view of knee for distal locking*
- *AP/angled HBL view of proximal femur for proximal locking*
- *AP/lateral view of knee for end-cap*

Procedure

- *Closed reduction is attempted by the surgeon manipulating the limb.* Traction can be applied by either the surgeon or assistant pulling the tibia distally. This positioning can be checked under X-ray with both AP and lateral views. If there is a multi-fragment fracture that requires reduction (e.g. a Y-shaped fracture separating the articular surface), then the fracture site will have to be opened for reduction and fixation via lag screws before nailing commences.

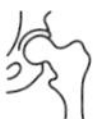

- *The C-arm is withdrawn while the limb is cleaned and draped once the manual reduction has been completed or abandoned in favour of open reduction.* While the C-arm is away from the patient as draping is taking place, it is often a good idea to wrap a nonsterile plastic bag over the X-ray tube, securing it with tape if necessary. This will protect the tube from blood spillage during the procedure, and make cleaning the machine at the end of the case much easier. The C-arm is covered by having a sterile drape placed over the receptor before it is brought back over the limb (Figures 13.5 and 13.6).

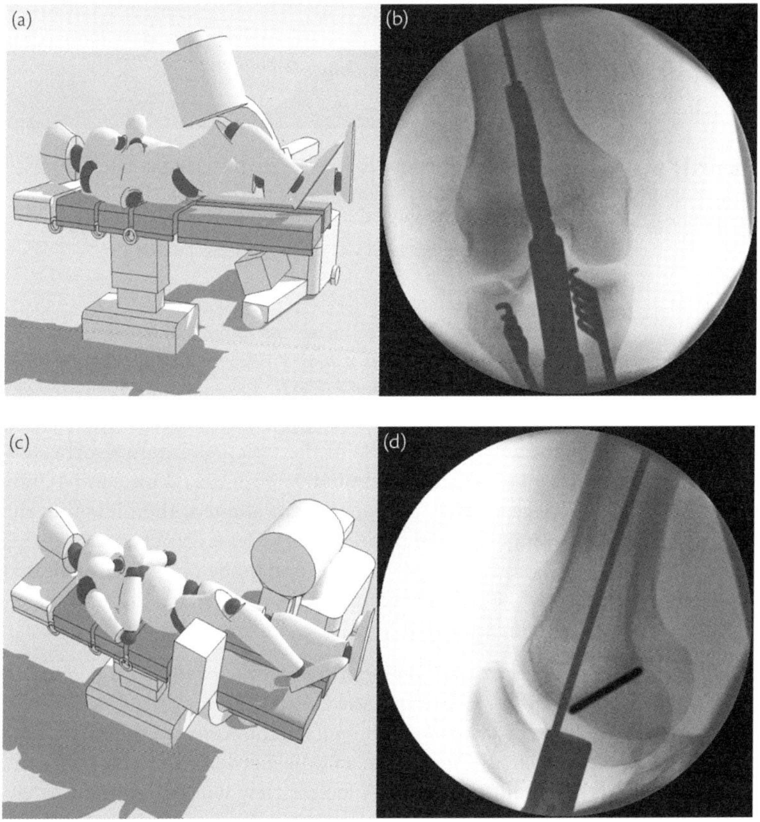

(a) (b) (c) (d)

Figure 13.5 Retrograde femoral nail insertion. (a) Anteroposterior view of right knee for intercondylar access. (b) Resulting image demonstrating drill over guidewire. (c) Horizontal beam lateral view of right knee. (d) Resulting image with guidewire anterior to Blumensaat's line (highlighted).

(b) and (d) Reproduced courtesy of Radiology Department, Leeds Teaching Hospitals NHS Trust, UK.

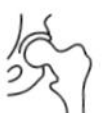

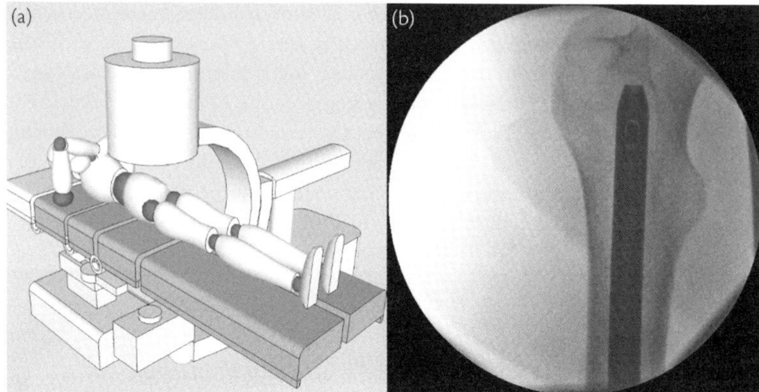

Figure 13.6 Locking for retrograde femoral nail. (a) Anteroposterior position for proximal locking. (b) Resulting image. Note: position of lesser trochanter allows assessment of rotation.

(b) Reproduced courtesy of Radiology Department, Leeds Teaching Hospitals NHS Trust, UK.

- *The surgeon may wish to use X-ray to check the alignment of the femur, by placing a radio-opaque object (such as a long guidewire) along the top of the femur, and imaging both the hip and knee in AP.* There should be a straight line between the middle of the femoral head and centre of the patella, continuing straight down the middle of the tibia. Alternatively, the surgeon may compare the affected and unaffected limbs. This can be done by rotating both legs so that the patellae are aligned, then imaging the hips in AP and comparing the position of the lesser trochanters. If this technique is used, it is imperative that the patient be positioned such that their pelvis is below the central column of the operating table, and the C-arm can centre over the affected hip.
- *The region around the patients' knee is then opened to allow access to the medullary canal. A short guidewire is inserted under X-ray control between the condyles of the knee into the medullary canal.* In the AP view, the entry point for the guidewire should be in the middle between the condyles, and in line with the medullary canal. A lateral view will be required to ensure that the wire is drilled into the 'safe zone' anterior to Blumensaat's intercondylar line, avoiding the cruciate ligaments. *Once the first guidewire is in place, the entry hole will be drilled out to allow access to the canal.*
- A long guidewire is inserted up the limb and across the fracture site into the proximal femur. *The position of the guidewire should be checked*

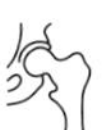

in AP views as it is advanced up the leg, with a lateral view performed once it appears proximal to the fracture site to ensure it has remained inside the medullary canal.

- Reamers of increasing size are now inserted over the guidewire, to widen the canal and allow insertion of the nail. As the limb is not held by the table support as in an antegrade nailing, the end of the limb may be pulled into traction by a member of the surgical team while the reamers are introduced. *Because of the risk of movement at the fracture site, imaging may be required to ensure the reamers cross over the fracture junction into the more proximal canal without diverting into the soft tissues or losing the reduction.*
- Once the canal has been reamed out sufficiently, the nail is inserted. As with other nailing procedures, *it may be necessary to image the fracture site during implantation to identify any loss of reduction due to the force of the nail being inserted.*
- Locking screws are inserted into the distal end of the nail. These are typically implanted via a guide attachment connected to the distal end of the nail itself. The drilling and implantation of the screws will be performed through the guide attachment, although the position and length of the screws will need to be checked under X-ray.
- *Due to the irregular shape of the distal femur and condyles, multiple views may be required to accurately demonstrate the position of the screws in relation to the anatomy.* This may include horizontal lateral, AP, and AP oblique views to show the angled medial or lateral borders of the condyles better. These images should be saved for archiving.
- *Proximal locking screws are inserted freehand under X-ray guidance, in the same manner as distal screws for an antegrade nail.* However, these screws may be inserted in the AP view. For long retrograde nails, positioning for a lateral view of the proximal nail holes can be very difficult, and may require adjusting the position of the patient's other leg. As before, *the screw holes must appear perfectly round and overlie each other before the screw can be inserted.* If AP screws are used, the C-arm will be in the AP position but *the receptor must be raised enough to allow the surgeon access to the anterior surface of the thigh.* Remember to make very fine adjustments when attempting to get the locking holes correctly aligned, as the long object–film distance will magnify all movements. *A second view will also be required once the screw is in place, to confirm its length in relation to the femur.* An HBL image angled up the femoral shaft should suffice for an AP screw, as long as it shows both cortices of the femur and the screw passing through them. One or two proximal locking screws may be used,

depending on the requirements of the case. Images of these in place (AP and laterals) should be saved for archiving.

- Finally, an end-cap is attached to the nail, to prevent bone growth into the nail. *Views of the knee will be required to demonstrate that the end-cap does not protrude into the articular surface of the knee joint. These images should be saved and archived to the PACS along with the dose information.*

13.5 Midshaft femoral plating

For periprosthetic fractures around a THR, or other injuries to the femoral midshaft where nailing is not feasible, a plate can be implanted onto the patients' femur as a fixation. This procedure allows direct visualization of the fracture and bony anatomy, and as such is not as reliant on imaging as other procedures.

Patient position

- Supine on traction table, with contralateral limb lowered and abducted

C-arm approach

- Between the patient's legs, at 90° to the affected femur, centred over the affected hip

Key imaging

- *AP/angled lateral views of fracture site*
- *AP view of hip for alignment check*
- *AP view of plate over fracture site*
- *AP view for measurement and insertion of screws*
- *AP view for insertion of cerclage wires (if used)*
- *AP/angled lateral views of plate*

Procedure

- *The fracture is manually reduced by manipulating the limb via the traction arm, with imaging used to check the position and alignment of the fracture site.* If closed manipulation via the traction arm proves unsuccessful, the middle of the thigh may be supported from underneath with a brace. *If a support is used, it is important that it be far enough from the fracture site to allow the C-arm to image the fracture, and for the radiographer to not strike it when moving the C-arm along the femur* (Figure 13.7).

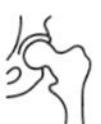

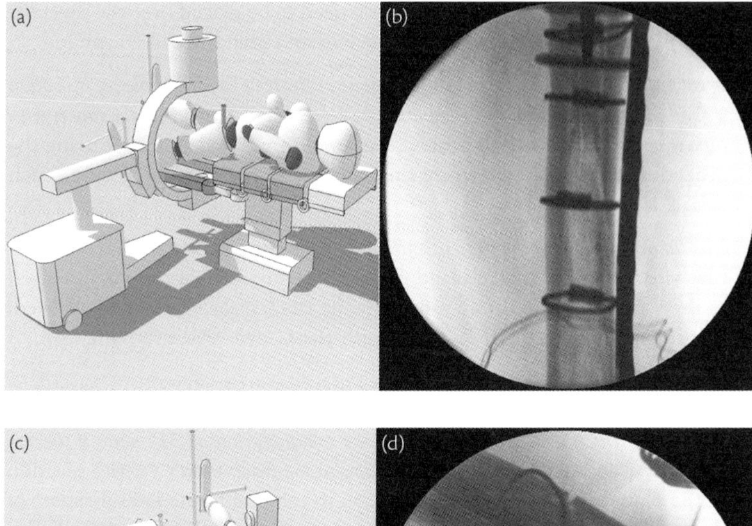

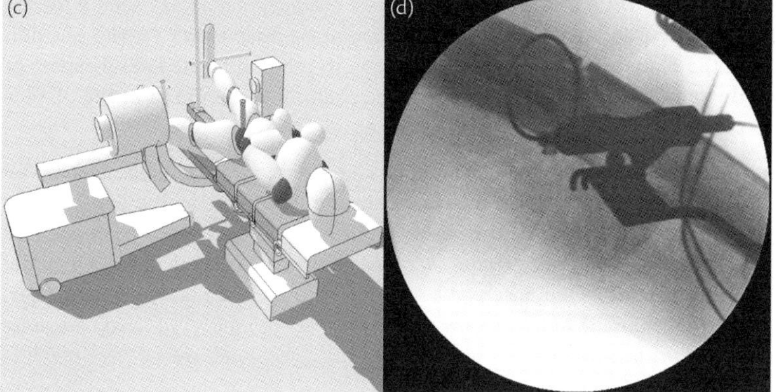

Figure 13.7 Plating of the right femur. (a) Anteroposterior positioning of R femur. Note L femur lowered to allow access. (b) Resulting image showing plate, cerclage wires. (c) Horizontal beam lateral positioning of R femur. (d) Resulting image showing cerclage wire being inserted around the stem of total hip replacement.

(b) and (d) Reproduced courtesy of Radiology Department, Leeds Teaching Hospitals NHS Trust, UK.

- Thee alignment of the femur will be checked under imaging. For this, *the views of the hip should include the entire femoral neck and hip joint, as well as both trochanters*. This allows the rotation of the leg to be judged correctly, and to avoid malrotation at the fracture site. Similarly, the fracture site will be checked for alignment and rotation.
- *The C-arm is withdrawn to allow cleaning and draping of the patient.* If a hanging drape is used as in a DHS, the C-arm receptor will not need to be

draped. Otherwise, a sterile drape will need to be placed over the receptor head before the C-arm is brought back in and imaging can continue.

- *While the C-arm is away from the patient as draping is taking place, it is often a good idea to wrap a nonsterile plastic bag over the X-ray tube, securing it with tape if necessary.* This will protect the tube from blood spillage during the procedure, and make cleaning the machine at the end of the case much easier.
- *The lateral margin of the patient's thigh is opened down to the femur.* The fracture site is located and reduced further if required. Clamps may be used to hold the reduction in alignment while the fixator is attached. If used, it is important not to strike these with the C-arm when moving around the leg.
- A plate is selected to be implanted. *The fit of the plate may be checked against the femur, which can be done under direct visualization or AP views if there is any uncertainty as to the plate in relation to the fracture site.* As the position of the plate can be seen by the surgeon in relation to the lateral aspect of the femur, a lateral view may not be required. Once the fit of the plate is satisfactory, it is attached to the femur.
- *A guide hole is drilled through the plate and across the cortices of the femur.* The depth of the hole is then measured through the plate with a depth gauge to assess the length of the screw required. *An AP view of the guide hole may be required at this point to check the position of the depth gauge.* Once the depth is established, a screw is inserted through the plate into the femur. *This procedure is repeated until there are sufficient number of screws on either side of the fracture site.*
- If there is a THR or other occlusion to the femoral canal in place, shorter screws may be inserted (that do not cross the medullary canal), or wiring may be inserted around the circumference of the femur to hold the plate to the bone. A curved hook is inserted around the femur, and a wire is fed through it. The hook is then brought over the wire and away from the femur, leaving the wire encircling the femur and plate. *AP views of the region demonstrating the wire on the bone may be required.* The wire is then tensioned, so that it grasps the plate against the femur. Once this is completed, *an AP view may be required to check the fit of the plate against the femur and the integrity of the surrounding bone*, as well as the position in relation to the tip of the THR (or whichever obstruction to the medullary canal is present).
- Once the plate is fully attached, *AP views demonstrating the full length of the plate and fracture site should be taken.* A lateral view of the fracture site and

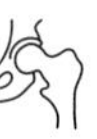

plate may also be required. *These images should be saved and archived to the PACS along with the dose information.*

References

Noordeen, M. H., Lavy, C. B., Briggs, T. W., and Roos, M. F. 'Unrecognised Joint Penetration in Treatment of Femoral Neck Fractures', *Bone and Joint Journal*, 75/B (1993), 448–49.

The Care of Patients with Fragility Fracture ('Blue Book')—British Geriatrics Society [WWW Document] (n.d.), http://www.bgs.org.uk/fallsresources-307/subjectreference/fallsandbones/bluebookfragilityfracture, accessed 4.26.17.

Salvi, A. E. 'The Chessboard Technique: A New Freehand Aiming Method for Rapid Distal Locking of Tibial Nails,' *Bulletin of the NYU Hospital for Joint Disease*, 66/4 (2008), 317–19.

14

Distal femur and knee

The knee is one of the main load-bearing joints of the body, and injuries to it can greatly reduce the functioning of the limb. These can involve damage to the joint or articular surfaces, or fractures to the long bones in case of high-energy trauma. The position of the contralateral leg can cause difficulty in positioning for imaging, but good positioning and technique should allow demonstration of the region for intervention.

14.1 Distal femoral plating

For supracondylar fractures or those where a femoral nailing would not be achievable, a plate and screws can be used as an extramedullary support. This may include cases where a total hip replacement (THR) or knee replacement (TKR) is in place that would prevent a nail insertion. A minimally invasive or an open approach may be used, depending on the nature of the fracture and limb. An open approach will require less imaging as the femur can be directly seen and manipulated by the surgeon; however, it will increase the risks of infection and blood loss due to the larger incisions required. A minimally invasive approach also results in smaller scars on the patient's limb.

Patient position

- Supine, with the affected limb horizontal and the contralateral limb raised or lowered to allow access

C-arm approach

- From the contralateral side at 90° to the affected femur, centred over the knee, and angled parallel to the femoral shaft

Key imaging

- *AP/lateral views superior to knee for closed reduction*
- *AP/lateral views of knee for compression screw (if used)*

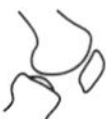

- *AP/lateral views for position and fit of plate*
- *AP view for drilling and screw insertion*
- *AP oblique view for screw position by medial condyle*
- *AP/lateral views of fracture site*

Procedure

- *Closed manipulation of the fracture is attempted by the surgeon.* Traction on the limb is used to manipulate the fracture back into anatomical reduction, and is checked under imaging. *Once the AP view is satisfactory, the C-arm is rotated under the table for a horizontal beam lateral (HBL) view.*
- *The C-arm is withdrawn while the area is cleaned and draped once the manual reduction has been completed or abandoned in favour of open reduction. While the C-arm is away from the patient as draping is taking place, it is often a good idea to wrap a nonsterile plastic bag over the X-ray tube, securing it with tape if necessary.* This will protect the tube from blood spillage during the procedure, and will make cleaning the machine at the end of the case much easier. The C-arm is draped by having a sterile drape placed over the receptor before it is brought back over the limb.
- *The region around the fracture site is opened.* If a compression screw is to be used (in the case of Y-shaped intra-articular fractures), it is implanted before the plate is attached to it. *A guidewire is inserted under imaging control in AP view through the condyles of the knee.* A lateral view may also be required to demonstrate the wire position in relation to the shaft of the femur. This wire is the guide for the condylar screw that will define the position and fit of the plate against the femur, and, as such, the position must be checked before the procedure continues (Figure 14.1)
- *Once the wire is in place, it is measured, and a cannulated drill or reamer is driven over it.* This may require imaging in the AP view to check the progress of the drill. The hole is then tapped, and the condylar screw is inserted.
- *A plate is inserted onto the lateral border of the femur, with the distal end of the plate positioned over the condylar screw.* The fit and position of the plate will be checked under X-ray in AP and lateral views; however, imaging may not be required here if an open approach has been used. The fracture site reduction will also be checked at this point.
- Once the plate is a satisfactory fit and the reduction has been achieved, the plate is secured to the bone at the site of the condylar screw. One or

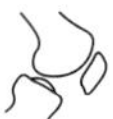

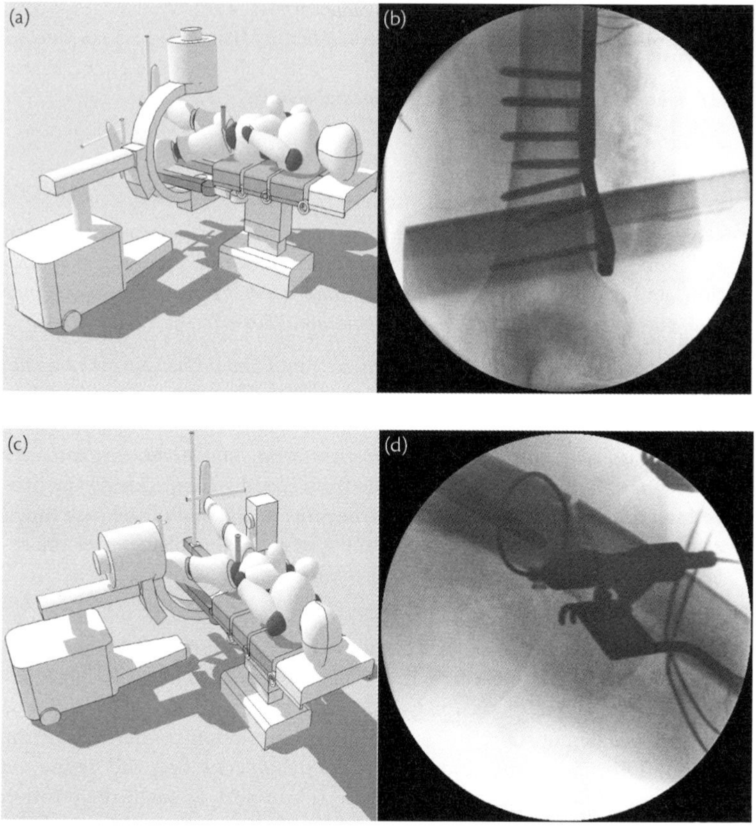

Figure 14.1 Distal plating of the femur. (a) Anteroposterior (AP) position for right knee. Note left leg lowered. (b) Resulting AP image with plate *in situ*. (c) Horizontal beam lateral position for right knee. (d) Resulting image (proximal) showing cerclage wire being implanted.

(b) and (d) Reproduced courtesy of Radiology Department, Leeds Teaching Hospitals NHS Trust, UK.

more smaller screws may also be implanted at the distal end of the plate to prevent rotation.

- *If a compression screw is not being used, once the reduction is satisfactory and any fragments are reattached with screws, a plate is inserted up from the knee along the lateral aspect of the femur.* The position and fit of this plate will need to be checked under AP views, with also a lateral view if required (especially in the case of minimally open procedures).

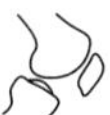

- Once the position of the plate is satisfactory, it is attached to the distal segment of the femur through the condyles. A drill guide is attached to the side of the plate, and guide holes are drilled through the plate's screw holes into the femur. *The position and depth of the drill may be checked under AP view.* The depth of the holes is then measured through the plate, and screws are inserted to fix the plate to the distal femur.
- The plate is attached to the proximal femur above the fracture site. Screw holes are drilled through the plate into the femur and measured before the correct-size screw is implanted, which affixes the plate to the femoral shaft. *AP views will be required to check the depth of the holes and fit of the screws as they are inserted.* Once sufficient number of screws have been implanted to maintain the fixation, final images of the implant and fracture site will be required.
- *AP and lateral views demonstrating the entire length of the implant and knee joint will be required, as well as possible AP oblique views to demonstrate the position of screws in relation to the medial epicondyle. These images should be saved and archived to the picture archiving and communication system (PACS) along with the dose information.*

14.2 Tension band wiring of patella

Transverse or stellate fractures of the patella typically require surgical intervention as flexing of the knee joint will pull the segments of the fracture apart. For transverse fractures, a tension band wiring (TBW) can be used. This technique distributes compressive force equally along the length of the fracture, rather than fixing at single points (e.g. with screws), which causes stress points that may fail and cause further damage.

Patient position

- Supine, with the affected knee flexed and supported

C-arm approach

- From the contralateral side at 90° to the femur, and centred over the affected knee

Key imaging

- *AP/lateral views for reduction*
- *AP/lateral views for insertion of K-wires*
- *AP/lateral/oblique views for tightening of wiring*

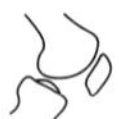

Procedure

- The region over the patella is cleaned, draped, and opened. The fracture is located and cleaned for fragments. The C-arm is draped and brought in at 90° to the patient's midline from the opposite side, so that the receptor is centred over the affected knee. *Lateral views are achieved by rotating the C-arm under the table to the HBL position.*
- *The fracture is manipulated into reduction and held with clamps.* These clamps will remain in place for the entire procedure, and it is important to avoid striking them with the C-arm receptor. AP and lateral views may be required at this point to check the reduction (Figure 14.2).
- *A K-wire is inserted axially (from top to bottom) into one of the fragment segments.* The K-wire is then driven across the fracture site and through the other segment. *The position of the wire will then be checked under X-ray in AP and lateral views, to ensure it crosses the fracture site securely and does not impinge on the articular surface.*
- *A second K-wire is then driven through the patella parallel to the first.* The position of the wire is checked in the same manner as the first.
- *A cable is wrapped behind the K-wires at one end, then brought down across the anterior surface of the patella.* It is then looped under the other ends of the K-wires and brought back up over the patella. This can be done either straight over the patella, or in a 'figure of 8' pattern, depending on the surgeon's preference. The K-wires are then trimmed at both ends and bent to hook around the cable.
- *The two ends of the cable are then twisted together.* This tightens the wiring and pulls the fracture segments into compression. *The reduction may be checked again in AP and lateral views as the cable is tightened.*
- Once the reduction is satisfactory, the ends of the cable are positioned so as to not damage the articular surfaces or the soft tissues around the knee. *Final AP and lateral views are then taken, with flexed or oblique views if required. These images should be saved and archived to the PACS along with the dose information.*

14.3 Cerclage wiring of patella

More complex stellate fractures of the patella with comminution can be treated with a wiring around the circumference of the patella. TBW, K-wiring, or screws may be used as well, depending on the complexity and position of the fractures.

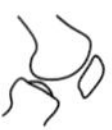

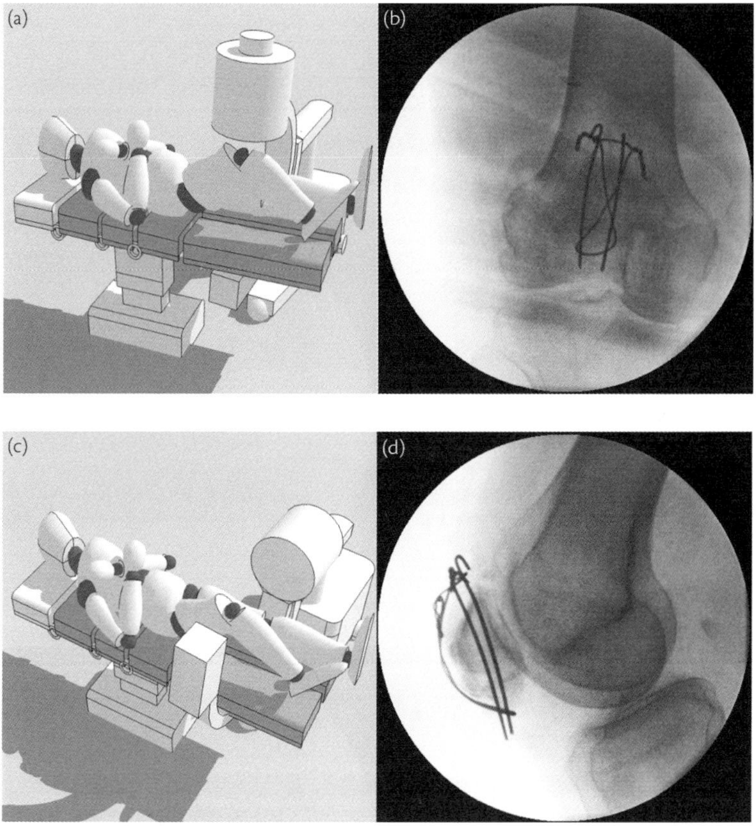

Figure 14.2 Patella. (a) Anteroposterior view of right patella. Note knee raised (under-knee support may be used). (b) Resulting image with tension band wiring *in situ*. (c) Horizontal beam lateral of right patella. (d) Resulting image.

(b) and (d) Reproduced courtesy of Radiology Department, Leeds Teaching Hospitals NHS Trust, UK.

Patient position

- Supine, with the affected knee flexed and supported

C-arm approach

- From the contralateral side at 90° to the femur, and centred over the affected knee

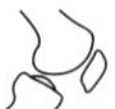

Key imaging

- *AP/lateral views of reduction*
- *AP/lateral/oblique views for tightening of wiring*
- *AP/lateral/oblique views of other fixators used*

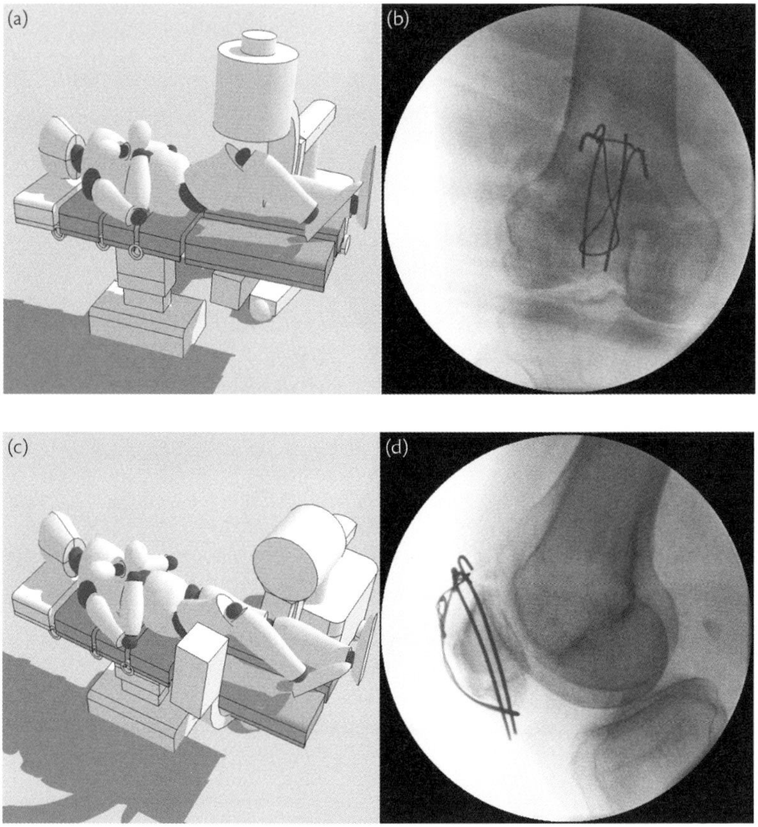

Figure 14.3 Wiring of patella. (a) Anteroposterior view of right patella. Note knee raised (under-knee support may be used). (b) Resulting image with tension band wiring *in situ*. (c) Horizontal beam lateral of right patella. (d) Resulting image.

(b) and (d) Reproduced courtesy of Radiology Department, Leeds Teaching Hospitals NHS Trust, UK.

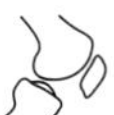

Procedure

- *The region over the patella is cleaned, draped, and opened.* The fracture is located and cleaned for fragments. The C-arm is draped and brought in at 90° to the patient's midline from the opposite side, so that the receptor is centred over the affected knee. *Lateral views are achieved by rotating the C-arm under the table to the HBL position.*
- *The fracture site is manually reduced and held in position with clamps.* These clamps will remain in place for the entire procedure, and it is important to avoid striking them with the C-arm receptor. AP and lateral views may be required at this point to check the reduction (Figure 14.3).
- *A cable is inserted around the superior edge of the patella, then fed around the border of the patella until it is fully encircled.* The ends of the cable are then twisted, to compress the fractures together. *AP and lateral views may be required during this process, to check the stability of the reduction and alignment of the fracture segments.* Once the compression from the cable is satisfactory, the ends of the cable are positioned so as to not damage the articular surfaces or the soft tissues around the knee.
- *Depending on the nature and complexity of the fracture, another fixation may be implanted, such as screws or TBW.* AP and lateral views of any additional fixation should be performed as and when needed (see section 14.2).
- *The final AP and lateral images, along with any flexed or oblique views performed to demonstrate the articular surfaces, should be saved and archived to the PACS along with the dose information.*

15

Tibia and ankle

The ankle and distal tibia can often be damaged through inversion injuries, or from twisting trauma at the foot. As a weight-bearing structure, it is important that the reduction allows the normal function of the limb to return as soon as possible.

15.1 Tibial plateau screws

Fractures to the tibial plateau will reduce the functioning of the limb and articulation of the knee, and, as such, will need to be reduced and fixated to stability if load-bearing through the limb is to be achieved. Often, it is the lateral side of the plateau that is damaged (from direct trauma to the lateral side of the knee causing excessive valgus angulation at the joint), the fixation of which will be covered here.

Patient position

- Supine, with the affected knee flexed and supported

C-arm approach

- From the contralateral side at 90° to the femur, and centred over the affected knee, with the angulation of the central ray parallel to the tibial plateau

Key imaging

- *AP/lateral views for reduction*
- *AP/lateral views for K-wire insertion*
- *AP/lateral views for screw insertion*

Procedure

- *The region over the proximal tibia is cleaned, draped, and opened.* The fracture is then manually reduced into anatomical position. Small incisions can be made to allow clamps to be placed onto the bone to aid and maintain

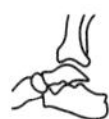

reduction. These clamps will remain in place for the entire procedure, and it is important to avoid striking them with the C-arm receptor.

- If minimally invasive reduction is not successful, the incisions can be widened to allow more direct manipulation of the fracture. *The position of the fractured segment and integrity of the plateau will be checked under AP and lateral views* (Figure 15.1).

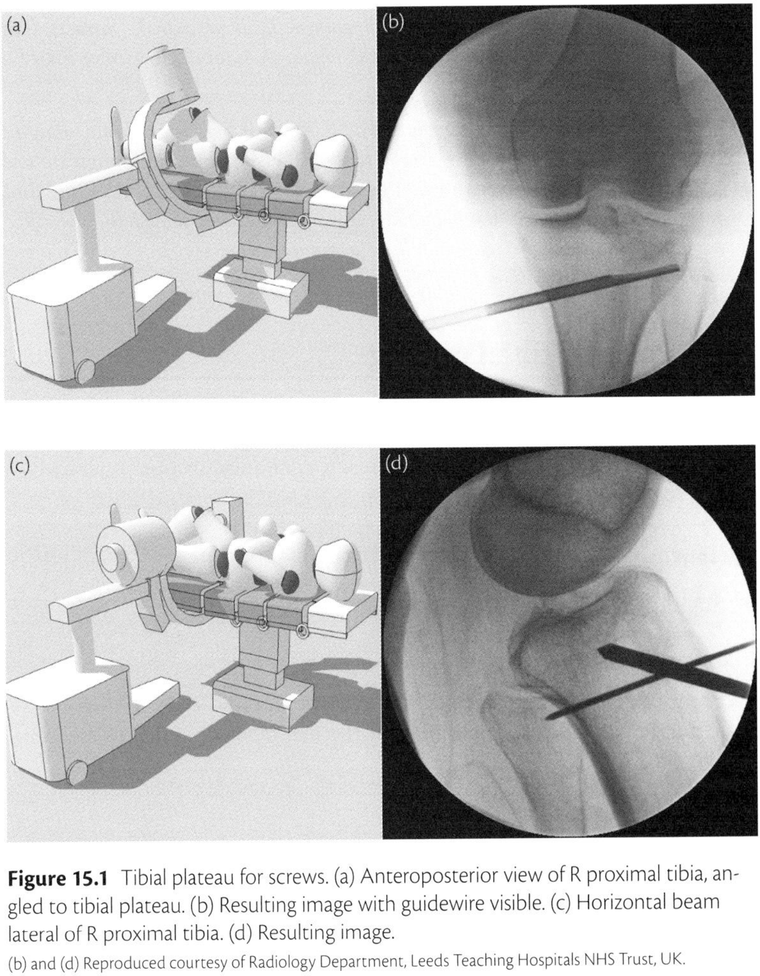

Figure 15.1 Tibial plateau for screws. (a) Anteroposterior view of R proximal tibia, angled to tibial plateau. (b) Resulting image with guidewire visible. (c) Horizontal beam lateral of R proximal tibia. (d) Resulting image.

(b) and (d) Reproduced courtesy of Radiology Department, Leeds Teaching Hospitals NHS Trust, UK.

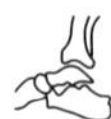

- *Once the reduction appears satisfactory, a temporary fixation may be made with K-wires.* These are inserted into the segment and across the fracture site into the tibia. *Their path may be checked under AP and lateral views as they are inserted.*
- *Lag screws can then be inserted across the fracture site to give full fixation.* The size and location of the fracture will determine how many screws are needed to secure and maintain the fixation. *In older patients or in those with longer fractures, a buttress plate may be placed onto the bone across the edge of the fracture before the screws are inserted through it.*
- *As the screws are inserted, their path within the bone and the reduction at the fracture site are checked under AP views.* A lateral view may also be required.
- *Once the fixation appears satisfactory, the K-wires and bone clamps may be removed and the final images can be taken.* These should demonstrate the screws (and plate if used) in full length, as well as the fracture site and knee joint in both AP and lateral views. *These views should be saved and archived to the picture archiving and communication system (PACS) along with the dose information.*

15.2 Proximal tibial plating

In cases of larger fractures or those that cross the shaft of the tibia, screws on their own may not be sufficient to maintain fixation and allow weight-bearing through the limb. In such cases, a plate may also be implanted to bridge across the fracture site.

Patient position

- Supine, with the affected knee flexed and supported

C-arm approach

- From the contralateral side at 90° to the femur and centred over the affected knee, with the angulation of the central ray parallel to the tibial plateau

Key imaging

- *AP/lateral views for reduction*
- *AP/lateral views for insertion and fit of plate*

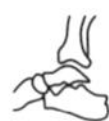

- *AP views for guide hole and screw insertion*
- *AP/lateral views for assessment of plate and fracture site*

Procedure

- *The region over the knee is cleaned, draped, and an incision made.* The fracture site is manually reduced. Small incisions can be made to allow

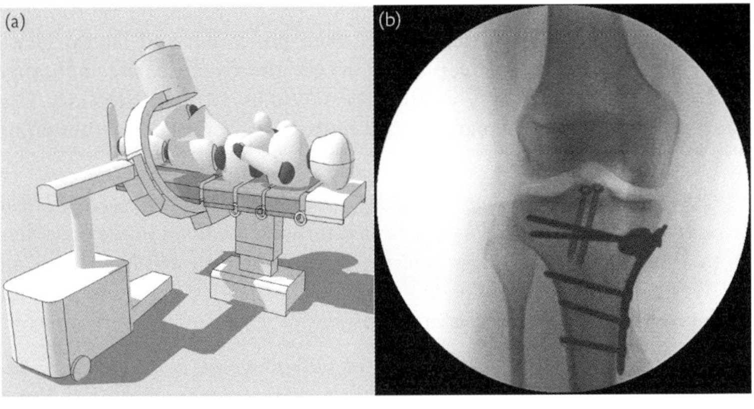

Figure 15.2 Tibial plating. (a) Anteroposterior view of R proximal tibia, angled to tibial plateau. (b) Resulting image. (c) Horizontal beam lateral view of R proximal tibia. (d) Resulting image demonstrating three-screw plate *in situ*.

(b) and (d) Reproduced courtesy of Radiology Department, Leeds Teaching Hospitals NHS Trust, UK.

clamps to be placed onto the bone to aid and maintain reduction. These clamps will remain in place for the procedure, and it is important to avoid striking them with the C-arm receptor.

- *AP and lateral views of the proximal tibia will be required to demonstrate the position of the fracture and anatomy, as well as the integrity of the tibial plateau at this point.* Once the reduction appears satisfactory, fixation may take place.
- *The plate is inserted through the incision site and placed on the border of the tibia.* The position may be checked under AP and lateral views to ensure that the plate reaches across the fracture site, and that there is sufficient space around the screw holes on either side. The fit and shape of the plate on the limb is also checked at this point (Figure 15.2).
- *Once the shape and position of the plate are satisfactory, it is affixed to the tibia with screws.* Guide holes will be drilled through the holes in the plate into the tibia before the screws, and the path of the drill will be checked in AP views. Once each guide hole is drilled, its depth is measured, and an appropriate-length screw is inserted.
- *Once sufficient number of screws are in place to maintain the reduction, the reduction clamps can be removed and the final images taken in AP and lateral views.* These should demonstrate the whole length of the implant and fracture site in both views. *These views should be saved and archived to the PACS along with the dose information.*

15.3 **Tibial nail**

Fractures of the shaft of the tibia may be fixated with an IM nail, in the same manner as those of the femur or humerus. However, due to the anatomy of the tibia and the need for access to the intramedullary canal via the knee, the positioning and technique differ from those of a femoral nailing. The use of a tibial nail allows the early mobilization of the patient, is more respectful to the surrounding soft tissues than a plate insertion, and helps avoid the risk of infections from the pins entering the skin that may occur with external fixators.

Patient position

- Supine, with the affected limb raised and flexed at the knee, and a radiolucent support under the knee

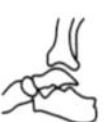

C-arm approach

- From the contralateral side at 90° to the tibia, and centred over the affected knee, with the angulation of the central ray parallel to the tibial plateau

Key imaging

- *AP/lateral views for fracture reduction*
- *AP/lateral views for opening of tibial plateau*
- *AP view of tibia for insertion of guidewire (with lateral view at fracture site)*
- *AP/lateral views for measurements*
- *Lateral views for insertion of distal locking screws*
- *AP/lateral views for position of end-cap, proximal locking screws, fracture site, and distal locking screws*

Procedure

- *The fracture is reduced manually under traction, and the position is checked under X-ray in AP and horizontal beam lateral (HBL) views.* If achieving or maintaining the reduction proves difficult, external clamps or a similar method may be used to hold the fracture in alignment after cleaning and draping. For oblique or complex fractures that cannot maintain alignment, further reduction may occur later in the procedure.
- *The C-arm is withdrawn while the patient is cleaned and draped.* A sterile drape will be placed over the receptor head of the C-arm before it can be brought back in over the patient.
- The region inferior to the patella is opened and the tibial plateau located. *A guide pin is inserted into the anterior edge of the tibial plateau to mark the entry point for the nail.* The position of the pin is checked under X-ray in AP and lateral views to ensure the point aligns with the medullary canal (Figure 15.3).
- Once the guide pin is in a satisfactory position, the entry point is opened with a cannulated drill. A guide wire is then inserted through the entry point and down through the medullary canal. *As the wire is inserted down the canal, the position should be checked under X-ray in AP view until it reaches the fracture site.*
- *Once the wire tip reaches the fracture site, traction may be applied to the limb again as the wire is progressed across the fracture into the distal tibia.* The limb

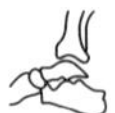

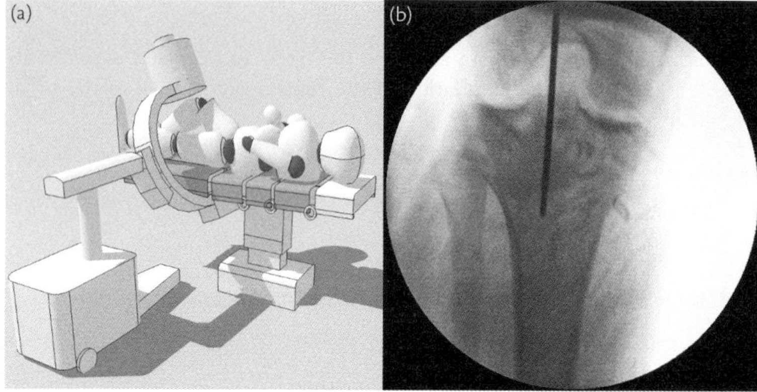

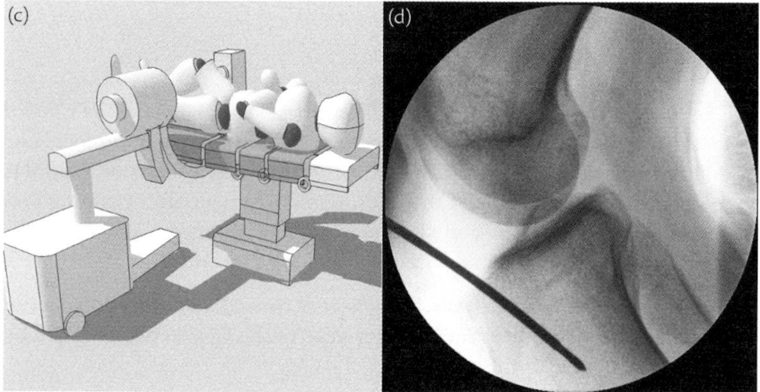

Figure 15.3 Insertion of tibial nail. (a) Anteroposterior view of the entry point of R proximal tibia. C-arm is angled to tibial plateau. (b) Resulting image showing guidewire being inserted. (c) Horizontal beam lateral view of R proximal tibia. (d) Resulting image showing guidewire advancing into medullary canal.

(b) and (d) Reproduced courtesy of Radiology Department, Leeds Teaching Hospitals NHS Trust, UK.

may be raised at this point to assist traction and reduction, and so the C-arm may be withdrawn to allow greater manipulation of the tibia.

- *Once the guidewire has crossed the fracture site, AP and lateral views will be required to ensure that the wire is within the distal medullary canal.* If the wire appears outside the canal in either view, it is withdrawn and reinserted across the fracture.

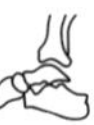

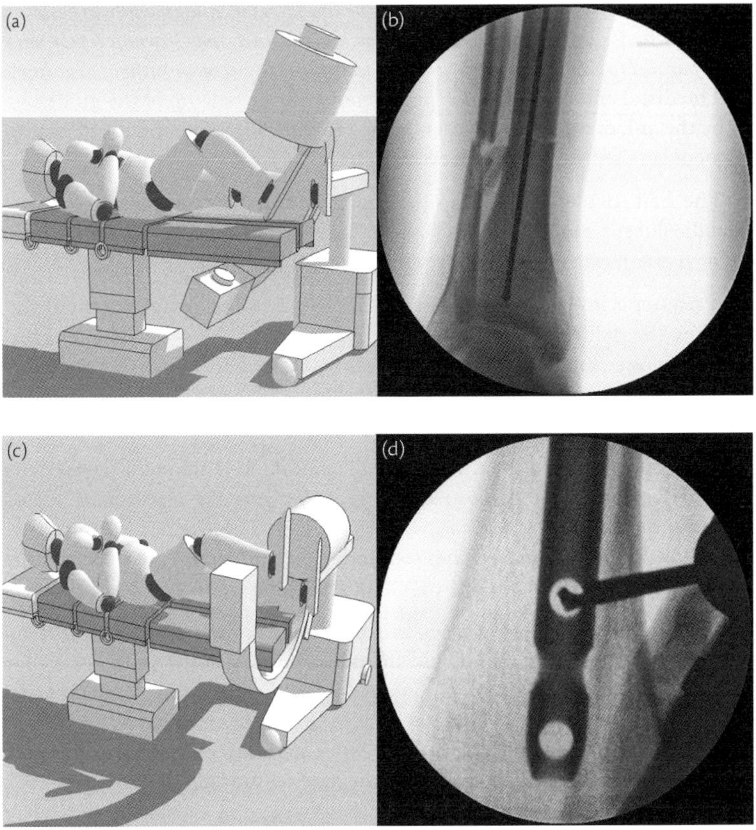

Figure 15.4 Distal tibial nail. (a) Anteroposterior view of R tibia. C-arm can be lowered as it is advanced towards ankle to lessen magnification. (b) Resulting image showing guidewire across fracture site. (c) Horizontal beam lateral view of R ankle, with limb supported above contralateral limb. (d) Resulting image of distal locking holes. Electronic magnification used here.

(b) and (d) Reproduced courtesy of Radiology Department, Leeds Teaching Hospitals NHS Trust, UK.

- The guidewire is progressed down towards the ankle joint. *The position of the end of the wire is checked in relation to the ankle joint under AP view* (Figure 15.4).
- The wire is measured to determine the length of the nail to be used. This can be done by measuring the length of the wire protruding from the tibial plateau and subtracting this from the full length of the wire. *Alternatively,*

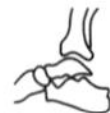

a radio-lucent ruler can be placed over the tibia, and measurements can be taken from it under AP view. If a radio-lucent ruler is used, the C-arm receptor must be parallel to the tibia, so as to give an accurate measurement without distortion. The distal end of the ruler is positioned over the ball-tip of the guidewire by the ankle; the C-arm is then moved to the knee joint, and the measurement is taken with an AP view.

- The nail diameter may also be established at this stage using another radio-lucent guide. *This will require both AP and lateral views, over the narrowest region of the medullary canal.*
- A reamer is inserted over the guidewire to widen the medullary canal and allow the nail to be inserted. *If the fracture is complex or unstable, imaging may be required at the fracture site as the reamer passes it, to ensure the reduction is not affected.* This process is repeated with larger-diameter reamers until the canal is of sufficient diameter.
- The nail is inserted from the tibial plateau on an alignment jig over the guidewire. *Imaging may be required at the fracture site to ensure the reduction is not affected as the nail passes through it.* The position of the distal end of the nail should be checked under AP and lateral views before the guidewire is removed and the locking screws inserted.
- The proximal locking screws are inserted through the alignment jig attached to the proximal end of the nail, and may not require X-rays for insertion. *The distal screws are inserted under X-ray control in lateral view. The C-arm is moved to the lateral view just proximal to the ankle, which may be raised on pads at this point to allow easier alignment of the C-arm and nail.* The distal locking holes are then identified on the lateral view.
- Electronic magnification can help demonstrate the holes and identify any misalignment. Collimation to the region around the locking holes (with both the linear and iris diaphragms) can greatly improve the image quality and reduce the backscatter dose to the surgeon while performing this view.
- *To demonstrate the locking holes correctly, the beam must be aligned directly through them, so that both sides are perfectly overlying.* Adjustments are made to the positions of both the C-arm and the leg to have the locking holes perfectly aligned on the image. *It is important to have the holes positioned as close to the centre of the receptor head as possible, as beam divergence will make true lateral alignment very difficult.* If the locking holes are not perfectly round in relation to the length of the nail, angling of the centre column can be used to improve alignment; if they are not perfectly circular

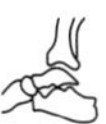

perpendicular to the length of the nail, slightly rotating the C-arm or the patient's leg can help correct the positioning (Figure 15.4).

- Once the C-arm and the nail-locking holes are exactly aligned, the surgeon will open the skin over the locking holes and align the drill to them. *Multiple images will be used to check that the point of the drill is directly over the locking holes. The C-arm and leg must remain entirely still during this process.* A screw hole is then drilled through the distal tibia and the nail holes by aligning the drill along the central ray, and the locking screw is inserted. *The procedure is then repeated for the second screw, often using the first as a guide for alignment.*
- Once the locking screws are in place, the alignment jig is removed and an end-cap is attached to the proximal end of the nail. *Final AP and lateral views should be taken of the proximal and distal ends of the nail, as well as of the fracture site. These images should be saved and archived to the PACS along with the dose information.*

15.4 Ankle fixation

Ankle fractures are very common, often caused by inversion injury or similar trauma. Depending on the nature of the trauma, they can involve up to all three malleoli, each of which may require its own fixation if stability at the ankle joint is to be restored. Each malleoli will be covered separately here.

Patient position

- Supine, with the affected ankle raised on a radio-lucent support if required

C-arm approach

- From the contralateral side at 90° to the tibia, and centred over the affected ankle
- Lateral views may be achieved by the surgeon rotating the limb, or an HBL view if required

Key imaging

- *AP/lateral views of ankle for reduction*
- *AP/lateral views of ankle for insertion of screws/wires*

Procedure

Lateral malleolus/distal fibula

- The region over the distal fibula is cleaned, draped, and opened to allow access to the fracture site. The fracture is located and manually reduced before fixation occurs.
- For oblique fractures of the distal fibula, a lag screw may be inserted across the fracture site. *A guide hole is drilled from the anterior edge of the fibula across the fracture site, and the hole measured.* A screw is then inserted through the hole and across the fracture site, and tightened so that it holds the fracture in compression. *AP and lateral views of the region may be required at this point to demonstrate alignment at the site or to document the position of the screw.*
- A plate is inserted onto the lateral border of the fibula, so that the middle region of the plate is over the fracture site. *The fit of the plate (including the number of screw holes above and below the fracture) may be checked under AP and lateral views. Clamps may be used to support the plate onto the bone, and it is important to avoid these when moving the C-arm around the limb.*
- Guide holes are drilled through the plate, and screws are inserted both superiorly and inferiorly to the fracture site to hold the plate in position. *AP views may be required for this to demonstrate the depth of the drill and screw into the patient's limb.*
- Once the position of the plate and screws appears satisfactory and the fracture appears stabilized, *AP and lateral views of the entire plate and ankle joint are taken. These images should be saved and archived to the PACS along with the dose information.*

Medial malleolus

- For the medial malleolus, the fracture is manually reduced and held with reduction clamps. *It is important to avoid these when moving the C-arm around the limb.*
- Guide wires are inserted up through the malleolus across the fracture site and into the tibia. *The position of the wires will need to be checked under AP and lateral views to ensure they are well sited in the bone and do not cross the articular surfaces.*
- By rotating the C-arm slightly over 90°, a true AP mortise view can be obtained to demonstrate the joint spaces without having to manipulate the limb.
- *Cannulated screws can then be driven over them to secure the reduction.* Alternatively, guide holes can be drilled and solid screws inserted.

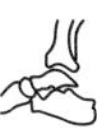

- *The position of the screws (either over the guide wires or in the pre-drilled guide holes) is checked in both AP and lateral views.* Once the appearance of the screws and fracture site is satisfactory, the guide wires and K-wires can be removed and the final images taken. *These images should be saved and sent to the PACS along with the dose report.*

Posterior malleolus

- The malleolus is manipulated back into anatomical position and checked under AP and lateral views if it cannot be directly visualized. A clamp may be used to hold the malleolus in reduction if required.

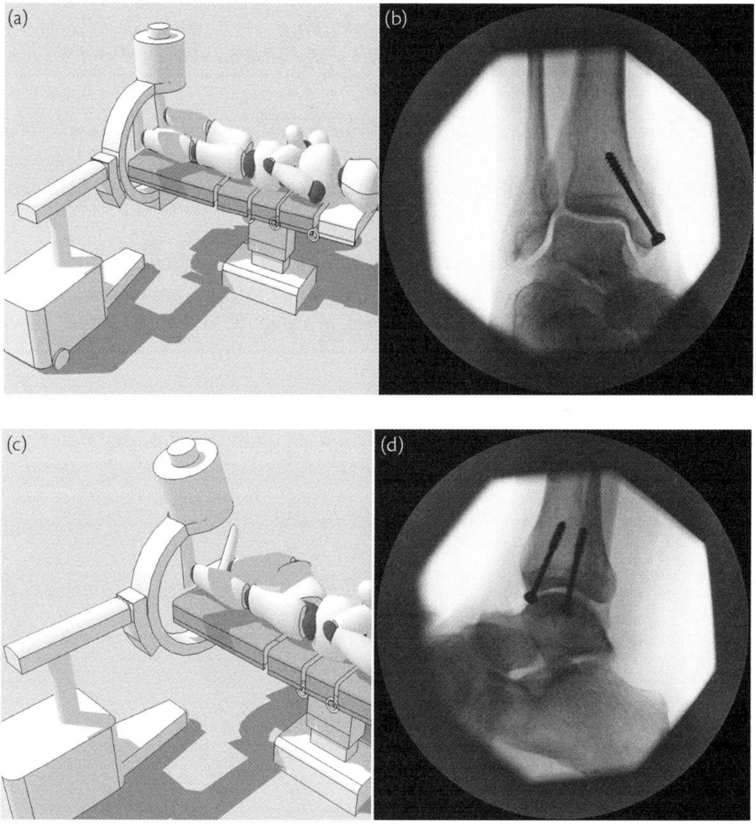

Figure 15.5 Right ankle positioning. (a) Anteroposterior view of R ankle supported on radio-lucent block. (b) Resulting image showing joint space, medial screws. (c) Lateral view of R ankle (note R leg externally rotated). (d) Resulting lateral image.

(b) and (d) Reproduced courtesy of Radiology Department, Leeds Teaching Hospitals NHS Trust, UK.

- *A guide wire is driven at around 90° to the fracture either from the anterior tibia or through the posterior malleolus, so that it crosses the fracture site. The position and depth of the wire will be checked under AP views as it is inserted.* Once the wire is in a satisfactory position, a second wire is inserted parallel to the first. *The position of this wire will also be checked under imaging, as will the reduction of the fracture.*
- Once the position of both wires is satisfactory, the wire outside the bone is measured and the screws to be inserted are selected. *A cannulated screw is inserted over each wire across the fracture site and tightened so as to hold the fracture firmly against the posterior tibia.*
- *Once both the screws are inserted, the guide wires can be removed. AP and lateral images of the ankle will be required to demonstrate the screw and fracture positions.* These images should be saved.
- *For more unstable fractures of the posterior malleolus, a buttress plate may also be inserted on the posterior tibia.* The plate is positioned over the fracture site at the posterior tibia. *Screw holes are then drilled through the plate into the tibial shaft, and the plate is fixed in position.*
- *Imaging in AP and lateral views will be required to check the position of the screws and plate, as well as the reduction at the fracture site.* These images should be saved. *Finally, all saved images should be sent to the PACS along with the dose report (*Figure 15.5*).*

16

Neurological procedures

Procedures for the correction or repair of damage to the nervous system can be daunting, and, in some centres, imaging for such cases may be performed only by more specialist radiographers. Here, a calm and methodical approach, combined with good communication with the surgical team, is the best technique to adopt.

16.1 Pedicle screws

Pedicle screws are used as anchor points to stabilize spinal injuries and correct misalignment or abnormal curvature of the spine. Once inserted, they can be attached to rods or frames that can release or apply pressure in directions as required to reduce the consequences of any vertebral pathology.

Patient position

- Prone, on radio-lucent table, with the region away from the tabular column

C-arm approach

- From the side opposite to the surgeon's approach, at 90° to the midline and centred over the affected region

Key imaging

- *AP/lateral views of spine to identify vertebral levels*
- *AP/AP oblique views of vertebra for insertion of guide/probe*
- *AP/lateral views of vertebra for depth and position of pedicle screw*
- *AP/lateral views of spine post-insertion of metalwork for checking reduction and position*

Procedure

- *The C-arm is draped and brought in from the side at 90° to the midline of the patient.* Typically, it will be rotated underneath the table for lateral view when required.

- The relevant vertebral level is identified before opening by prominent landmarks and palpation of the spinous processes. *Alternatively, imaging in AP view can be used to count the relevant levels from a landmark.*
- The region around the site is opened, and the insertion point at the pedicle is found. The bone cortex is cut away, and a guidewire or probe is inserted through the pedicle entry point into the vertebral body. This creates a path for the screw to be inserted into.

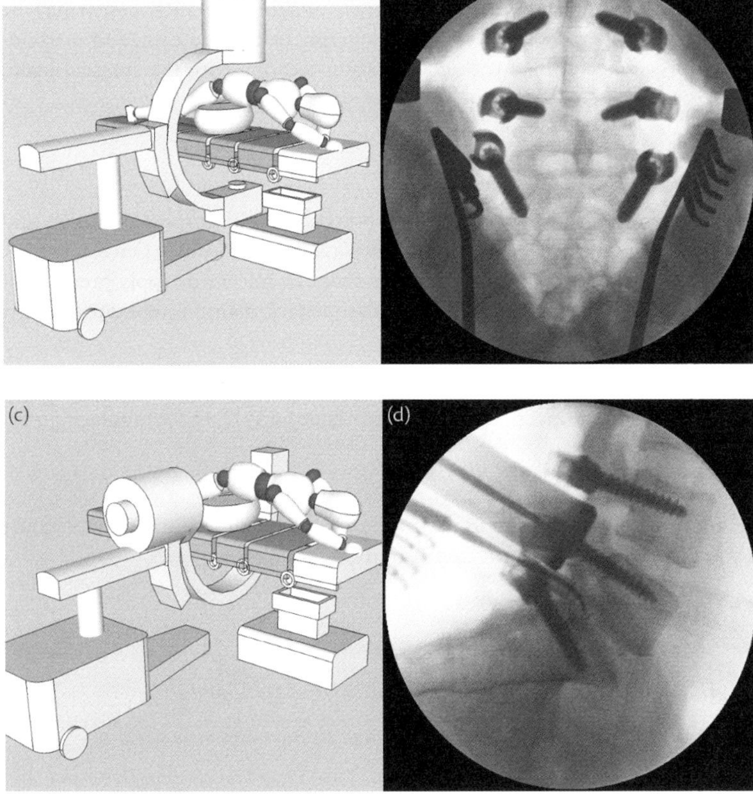

Figure 16.1 L4-S1 pedicle fixation. (a) Anteroposterior view of lumbar spine. (b) Resulting image, with pedicle screws in L3–L5 bilaterally. Note tissue retractors. (c) Horizontal beam lateral position of lumbar spine, under-table rotation of C-arm. (d) Resulting image showing pedicle screws in place.

(b) and (d) Reproduced courtesy of Radiology Department, Leeds Teaching Hospitals NHS Trust, UK.

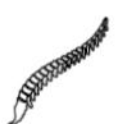

- *Imaging is required either in AP view only (Sethi et al. 2012), or AP and lateral views (Puvanesarajah et al. 2014) as the probe is inserted, depending on the surgeon's preference.* Angling the C-arm into a slight AP oblique so that the central ray is along the path of the probe can demonstrate the path in relation to the spinal canal (Ramis 23:49:48 UTC).
- *Linear collimation parallel to the spine should be used to cut down on scatter and dose* (Figure 16.1).
- By angling the central ray to the curvature of the region in the AP view (aligning to the end plates of the vertebral body), the vertebra can be demonstrated in profile (Betz et al. 2017).
- *Screws will be inserted typically at multiple levels above and below the site of pathology.* The receptor head may need to be raised to allow access to the surgeon.
- *Once the guide hole has been created, the screw is inserted. Images may then be taken to confirm and document the position of the screw.* The process is then repeated for the pedicle on the opposite side and at the other required levels.
- Once inserted, the screws may be attached to rods or other hardware. *AP and lateral images are required, once completed, to check reduction/decompression and spinal alignment, as well as the fit of the implanted hardware. These images should be saved and sent to the picture archiving and communication system (PACS) along with the dose report.*

16.2 **Anterior plating**

Damage to the cervical spine may be repaired by implanting a plate onto the anterior surfaces of the cervical bodies. This may be combined with pedicle screws or other fixators to add stability to the spine.

Patient position

- Supine on radio-lucent table, with head and neck supported on extension

C-arm approach

- From the side opposite to the surgeon's approach, at 90° to the midline and centred over the affected region

Key imaging

- *Lateral view of spine to identify vertebral levels*

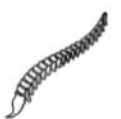

- *Lateral/AP views for insertion of distractors or other traction implants*
- *Lateral/AP views for fit and contouring of plate*
- *Lateral view of spine for insertion of fixation screws*

Procedure

- *The C-arm is draped and brought in from the side at 90° to the midline of the patient.* It is then rotated to the lateral position (Figure 16.2).
- *The level of injury is located through horizontal beam lateral (HBL) images.* The region is then opened.
- The damaged bone and cartilage are cleaned away. A distractor may be inserted into the vertebral body above and below, to separate the damaged region and allow access. *Lateral images may be required as these are inserted.*
- Bone graft or prosthesis may be inserted if enough of the cervical body is removed or damaged. *The fit and position of these may be checked through AP and lateral images.*
- The plate is applied to the spine and contoured to fit. *The position and fit of the plate is checked in AP and lateral views.*
- *Screw holes are drilled through the plate under lateral imaging to check their depths.* AP views may also be required if there is any uncertainty as to the path of the screw holes.

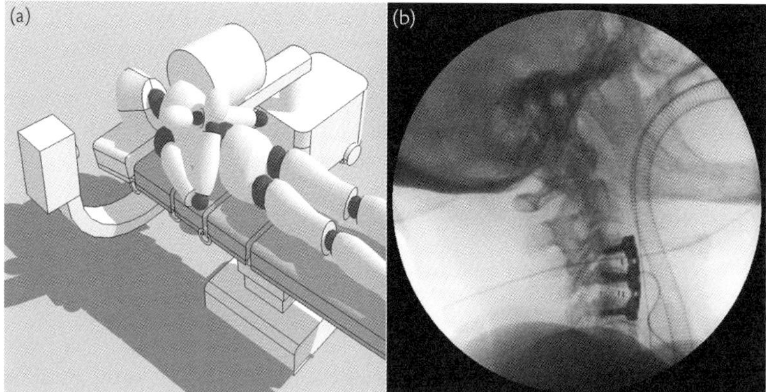

Figure 16.2 Anterior plating of C3–C5. (a) Lateral C-spine approach. Note receptor head closer to body to reduce magnification. (b) Resulting image showing C3–C5 plate *in situ*.

(b) Reproduced courtesy of Radiology Department, Leeds Teaching Hospitals NHS Trust, UK.

- *Screws are then inserted and positioned under AP and lateral views. Once the fit of the plate appears satisfactory, final views are taken. These should be archived to the PACS along with the dose report.*

References

Betz, R., Lonner, B., and Shah, S. [WWW Document], *X-Ray Imaging and Targeting* (2017), https://www.depuysynthesinstitute.com/spine/qs/DSUSSPN12151123c, accessed 5.30.17.

Puvanesarajah, V., Liauw, J. A., Lo, S., Lina, I.A., and Witham, T. F. 'Techniques and Accuracy of Thoracolumbar Pedicle Screw Placement', *World Journal of Orthopedics*, 5/2 (2014), 112–23. doi:10.5312/wjo.v5.i2.112.

Ramis, H., 23:49:48 UTC. Technique transpedincular screw placement. (n.d.), https://www.slideshare.net/RamisHuseynov/techniquetoinsert.

Sethi, A., Lee, A., and Vaidya, R. 'Lumbar Pedicle Screw Placement: Using Only AP Plane Imaging', *Indian Journal of Orthopaedics*, 46/4 (2012), 434–38. doi:10.4103/0019-5413.98832.

17

Paediatrics

As children's bones are still growing, different techniques are employed for the reduction and fixation of fractures in children than those used in adults. For example, their bones must not be damaged or impinged upon in a way that will affect further growth. Similarly, there are injuries that can affect the growth plates (Salter–Harris injuries), which are not present in adult trauma, and these may be treated differently to fractures of mature bone. For all paediatric procedures, radiation protection is of paramount significance. This is best achieved by using dose reduction settings on the image intensifier (II), good collimation to avoid excessive irradiation, and judicious use of Pb shielding on or around the patient.

17.1 Manipulation under anaesthesia (MUA)

Some fractures can be reduced to anatomical stability by manipulation of the limb without opening the area. This has the advantage of minimizing the risk of infection and scarring, as the skin is never broken. For these procedures, the C-arm can often be rotated, such that the limb is placed upon the receptor. This minimizes magnification and dose, while improving image quality. However, remember that the resulting image will appear reversed on the monitors, and the receptor head must be covered with a drape, especially when plaster is being applied. Also remember that, if the reduction is not successful, and wiring or plating is required, the limb *must* be moved onto a radio-lucent support, and the C-arm returned to the under-couch–tube position. Any mistakes while drilling or inserting wires with the limb supported on the receptor head will, at best, damage the C-arm, and, at worst, endanger the patient, surgeon, and radiographer (Waseem and Kenny 2000).

As usual, the position of the fracture will need to be seen in multiple views to check alignment and stability, and then rechecked once plaster has been applied as a fixator. Typically, the surgical team will manipulate the limb into the required position without the need for adjusting the C-arm positioning. However, some adjustment may be required for images after plaster casting

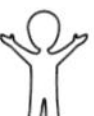

is applied (e.g. above-elbow casts will require adjustment to the C-arm to allow a lateral wrist view).

Post-reduction and post-plaster views (both AP and lateral) of the limb (plus any other stress views as required by the surgical team) should be saved and archived to the picture archiving and communication system (PACS) along with the dose information.

If the reduction cannot be made stable on its own, internal fixation may be used to support the fracture in position for healing. K-wires will often be used as a fixation (such cases are often booked as 'MUA +/− K-wiring').

17.2 K-Wiring

K-wires can be used as a minimally invasive internal fixator for paediatric fractures. Typically, the fracture will be manually reduced, as in an MUA, before wires are inserted through very small skin incisions. As with all internal fixations that cannot be directly visualized, imaging will be required to check the position of the wires and fracture. This will be required with the limb supported on a radio-lucent support (*never use the receptor head as a support during any procedure involving the implantation of fixators*) (Waseem and Kenny 2000), with the receptor head over the limb in a sterile drape.

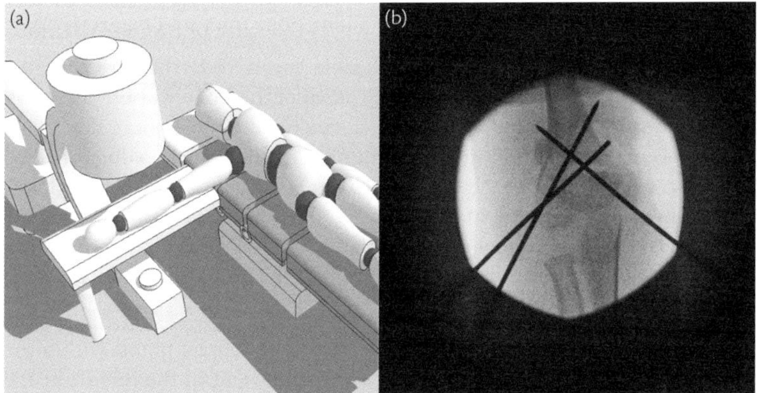

Figure 17.1 Paediatric elbow K-wiring. (a) Anteroposterior (AP) view of elbow in supine position. (b) K-wires inserted through elbow condyles into humerus in AP position.
(b) Reproduced courtesy of Radiology Department, Leeds Teaching Hospitals NHS Trust, UK.

Once the MUA has been completed, AP and lateral views may be used to demonstrate the entry point of the wire in relation to the anatomy before a small incision is made and the wire is driven into the bone. The progress of the wire across the fracture site will also be checked in AP and lateral views. The number of wires to be inserted will vary, depending on the fracture site and the stability of the reduction.

Once all the wires have been adequately sited, AP and lateral views demonstrating the fracture site and fixation (along with any stress views or others required by the surgeons) should be taken and saved. Post-plaster views may also be required once the wire sites are dressed and casting applied. These should also be saved, and the saved images must be archived to the PACS along with the dose information (Figure 17.1).

17.3 Elastic nailing for long bones

For paediatric long bone fractures, the standard treatment is closed reduction with casting. However, where the reduction cannot be maintained or other factors are present, surgical intervention may be required.

When implanting an IM nail into a long bone, the insertion point for the nail is typically drilled across a growth plate. For fully grown adult patients whose plates have fused, this is not an issue. However, with paediatric patients, such damage to the plate may cause growth issues in the bone. As an alternative to implanting an IM nail or plate to support the reduction, 'elastic stable intramedullary nails' (ESINs), also known as 'titanium elastic nails' (TENs), may be used to support a long bone fracture (Figure 17.2).

These implants consist of curved, flexible metal rods that are inserted through small holes into the medullary canal of the bone without affecting the epiphysis. Once in place, they act as flexible internal splints that allow some movement at the fracture site while holding the bone in reduction. The advantages of this system include the avoidance of damage to growth plates, smaller incisions resulting in less scarring and soft tissue damage than IM nails or plates, promotion of callus formation at the fracture site by allowing limited movement, and earlier mobilization of the limb (Sankar et al. 2007; Swindells and Rajan 2010).

The curve of these nails means each one has three contact points within the medullary canal (at the proximal and distal ends, and in the middle at the apex of the curve). A single nail may be inserted, typically, for fractures of the radius or ulna; or, in larger bones with wider canals, two nails can be inserted. By aligning the two nails so that their curves oppose each other,

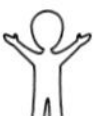

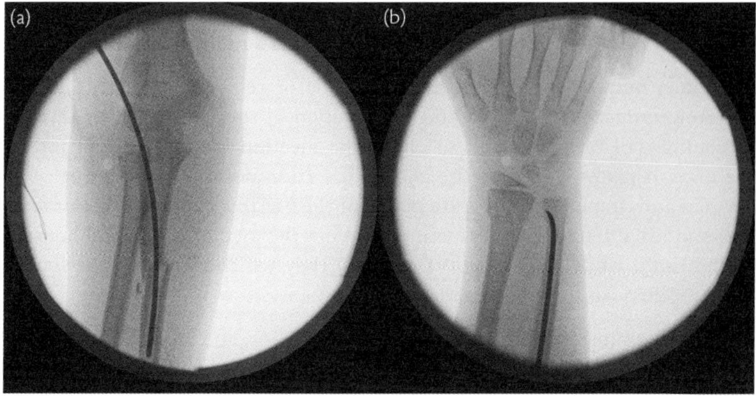

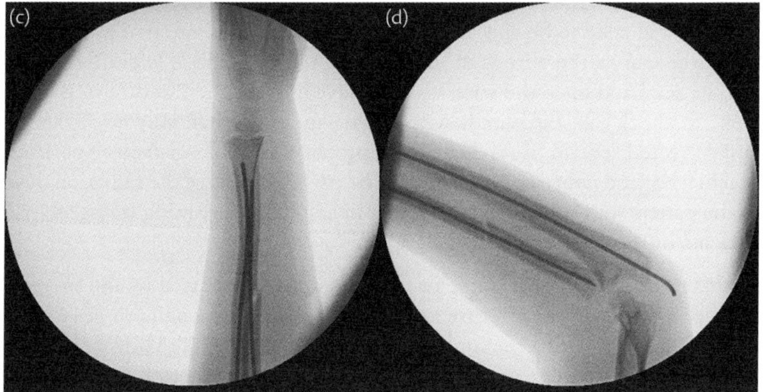

Figure 17.2 Elastic nailing of radius and ulna. (a) Flexi-nail being inserted into the proximal ulna crossing the fracture site. (b) Distal end of the nail in distal ulna. (c) Lateral image demonstrating nails in both radius and ulna. (d) Lateral view of proximal nails. Note protrusion for ease of removal.

Reproduced courtesy of Radiology Department, Leeds Teaching Hospitals NHS Trust, UK.

the system gives support to the limb and prevents misalignment or rotation at the fracture site.

The patient is placed supine on the table, with the affected limb positioned to allow access and imaging. For femoral fractures, the unaffected leg is flexed and abducted to allow the C-arm access between the patient's legs. For tibial fractures, the affected tibia is raised slightly on a radio-lucent support, while, in upper limb fractures, the limb is supported on a radio-lucent arm board.

The nails may be inserted either antegrade or retrograde, depending on the area undergoing fixation and the position of the fracture. Preliminary screening will be performed to check the location of the fracture and of the growth plates closest to the chosen insertion point. Once the region is cleaned and draped, incisions are made for the nail insertion points. For femoral and tibial fractures, these will be on both the medial and lateral borders of the limb, while, in humeral fractures, they will both be on the lateral border, one positioned superior to the other.

A nail is then inserted through the first entry point, and advanced along the bone. The position of the end of the nail will be checked under imaging, until it crosses the fracture site. As there is no guidewire used in this procedure to maintain the reduction and guide the implants, the reduction of the fracture will need to be checked under X-ray (with the limb manipulated by the surgeons) as the wire is driven across. At this point, a lateral view will also be required once the wire looks to have crossed the fracture in the AP view, to check that the wire is within the canal. The nail may be advanced and retracted several times during this process before a satisfactory position is achieved, and hence collimation may be useful to reduce the radiation dose to the patient and surgeons. Remember to avoid live screening for paediatric patients unless absolutely necessary.

An external radio-lucent frame or manipulator may be used by the surgeon to help manipulate the fracture site into reduction as the nail crosses it. It is important not to strike the limb or frame while moving the C-arm from AP to lateral, or to interfere with the reduction in any way. Alternatively, traction may be applied to the limb by the surgeons to aid the reduction. Once the nail appears within the canal in both views, it is advanced towards the epiphysis and the position checked under AP view. The nail may be trimmed to size at this point to prevent excessive protrusion at the entrance site, which will impinge on the surrounding tissues (Salonen et al. 2014). The second nail (if one is used) is then inserted in the same manner.

If a second nail is inserted, once it is in place, it may be rotated within the canal, so that the curves of the nails mirror each other. Once the position is satisfactory, AP and lateral views of the full length of the nails are required, particularly demonstrating the three contact points per nail, the depths of the ends of the nails in relation to the growth plates, and the entry points. The reduction of the fracture site will also be checked under at least two views. These images should be saved and archived to the PACS along with the dose information (Synthes 1998).

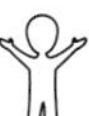

References

Salonen, A., Lahdes-Vasma, T., Mattila, V., Välipakka, J., and Pajulo, O. 'Pitfalls of Femoral Titanium Elastic Nailing', *Scandinavian Journal of Surgery*, 104/2 (2014), 1–6.

Sankar, W., Jones, K., Horn, B., and Wells, L. 'Titanium Elastic Nails for Pediatric Tibial Shaft Fractures', *Journal of Children's Orthopaedics*, 1/5 (2007), 281–86.

Swindells, M. and Rajan, R. 'Elastic Intramedullary Nailing in Unstable Fractures of the Paediatric Tibial Diaphysis: A Systematic Review', *Journal of Children's Orthopaedics*, 4/1 (2010), 45–51.

Synthes. *The Titanium Elastic Nail System: Technique Guide*, Synthes (USA, 1998).

Waseem, M. and Kenny, N. W. 'The Image Intensifier as an Operating Table—A Dangerous Practice', *The Journal of Bone and Joint Surgery*, 82/January (2000), 95–96.

18

Urology

Most urology procedures requiring imaging involve removing or bypassing any occlusions to the flow of urine from the kidneys. This may be performed by implantation of ureteric stents that provide a patent channel for urine flow from the renal pelvis to the bladder, removal of occlusions (typically stones) by either extraction or lithotripsy, or implantation of an external stoma that drains urine from the renal pelvis. For demonstrating the urinary tract under X-ray, an iodine-based contrast is used. This may be administered through a catheter into the ureter or renal pelvis, or dispensed percutaneously into the kidney to demonstrate the anatomy and outflow. The radiation dose may be higher in urological procedures than in orthopaedic cases due to the thickness of the patient's abdomen as compared to the extremities, and the need for longer screening times to demonstrate the flow of the contrast agent. As with any imaging procedure involving the pelvis and abdomen, where women of child-bearing age are being operated upon, it is essential to confirm negative pregnancy status before proceeding with the operation, and to document the pregnancy status in the operative notes or radiology systems.

18.1 Retrograde pyelogram

Patient position

- Supine, on a radio-lucent table, with legs separated in supports, hips brought to the end of the mattress, and arms over the chest; the patient's kidneys (roughly at the level of the elbow when arms are by the side) to be positioned below the centre column of the table

C-arm approach

- At 90° to the patient's midline from whichever side is the most practical, and centred over the patient's bladder, with space to move up to the kidneys without striking the patient's arms

Key imaging

- *AP view of bladder for catheterizing of ureter(s)*

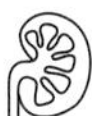

- *AP view of ureter(s) and kidney(s) for positioning of guidewires and other hardware*
- *AP view of ureter(s) and kidney(s) filled with contrast to demonstrate patency and flow*

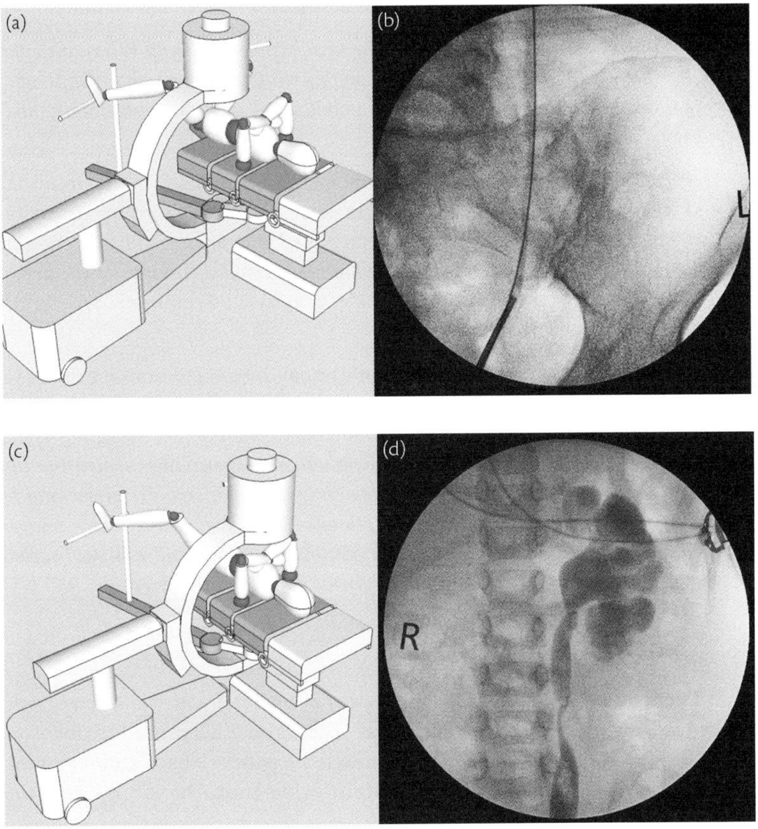

Figure 18.1 Retrograde pyelogram. (a) Positioning over bladder from left side. (b) Resulting image of left distal ureter cannulated with guidewire. (c) Positioning over left kidney. Note arms raised onto chest. (d) Image of left kidney with contrast and guidewire. Linear collimation may be of use here.

(b) and (d) Reproduced courtesy of Radiology Department, Leeds Teaching Hospitals NHS Trust, UK.

Procedure

- A scope is fed into the patient's bladder, and the ureter of the side under investigation is cannulated. *With the C-arm centred over the bladder, follow the guidewire or flow of contrast up the ureter while screening in AP view.*
- Pulsed exposure settings will lower the radiation dose to the patient and theatre staff, but will blur movement of structures such as guidewires, and, as such, should be used sparingly. *Linear collimation parallel to the ureters can be used to reduce radiation dose and improve image quality.*
- *If contrast is being used to visualize the ureters, images should be saved as the ureters fill, demonstrating their entire length from bladder to kidney.* Similarly, any images demonstrating the renal pelvis filled with contrast should also be saved.
- If a stent is being implanted, it is important to demonstrate the proximal end within the kidney to ensure it is in place and secured. *Many stents feature ends that curl once the guidewire is removed to secure them in position, and so images should be saved once the wire has been removed.* Images of the proximal end of the stent within the bladder may also be required, depending on the preference of the surgeon.
- For lithotripsy procedures, a wire or optical fibre is fed up the ureters to the position of any stones, to break them into passable fragments. This is often done under direct scope control; however, the position of the scope can be checked under screening. *Another injection of contrast at the end of the procedure can be used to demonstrate flow down the ureter and to identify any other obstructions or locations of stone fragments. These images should be saved and archived to the picture archiving and communication system (PACS) along with the dose information* (Figure 18.1).

18.2 Antegrade pyelogram

For patients with renal blockages that cannot be dealt with via a retrograde procedure, an antegrade pyelogram may take place. This procedure involves accessing the kidney percutaneously though the patient's back and removing occlusions or implanting a tube to drain urine from the kidney into the bladder or an external site.

Patient position

- Prone, on a radio-lucent table, with the upper abdomen away from the centre column of the table
- Legs separated and supported

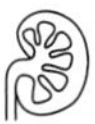

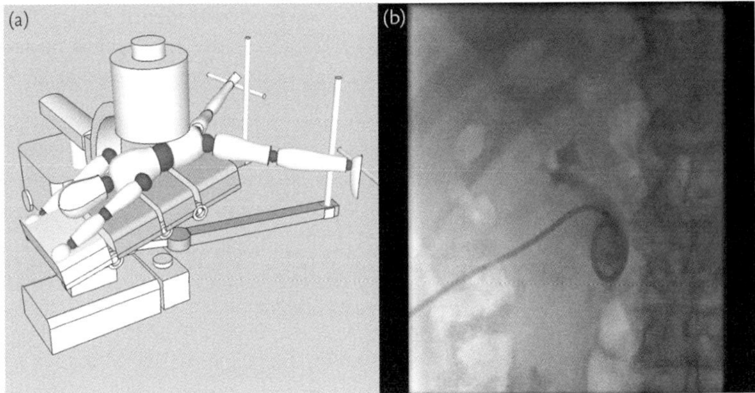

Figure 18.2 Antegrade percutaneous pyelogram. (a) Prone position for access to urinary tract and percutaneous access to kidney. (b) Resulting image showing renal pelvis filling with contrast through catheter.

(b) Reproduced courtesy of Radiology Department, Leeds Teaching Hospitals NHS Trust, UK.

C-arm approach

- At 90° to the patient's midline, from the opposite side to the kidney under investigation

Key imaging

- *AP view of bladder to check the position of catheter and guidewire*
- *AP view of ureter to kidney with contrast to locate the renal pelvis*
- *AP view of ureter to check the position of stent (if used) or flow of contrast from kidney to bladder*

Procedure

- The patient is laid prone on a radio-lucent table, with legs separated and supported.
- The C-arm is draped and brought in at 90° from the opposite side of the patient to allow the surgeon access (Figure 18.2).
- A scope is fed into the patient's bladder and the ureter catheterized. Contrast will be fed up the ureter to highlight the renal pelvis. *AP imaging should be used to follow this flow up to the kidney.*

- Once the renal pelvis is identified, the surgeon will identify the point at which they will open the soft tissues to access the renal pelvis under screening. *Once the entry point is found, the C-arm can be pulled back to allow easier access.*
- Once the renal pelvis has been accessed, a stent may be fed down towards the bladder, or an external catheter may be fitted. Alternatively, stones within the kidney can be directly broken up or removed.
- Images may be required at the end of the case to check the positioning of any implants and to ensure the free drainage of contrast. *These should be saved to the PACS along with the dose information.*

19

Hepatobiliary

Pathology of the gall bladder or biliary tree may be treated surgically if required. This can involve the removal of stones and occlusions from biliary ducts, opening up of the ducts where they have become narrowed, or removal of the gall bladder itself if required. These procedures are often performed under a minimally invasive approach to reduce the risks of infection and scarring, and as such can require imaging guidance (Cotton and Williams 2011).

19.1 Laparoscopic cholangiogram

For patients with gallstones or other gall bladder conditions, a cholecystectomy may be performed. This procedure involves the removal of the gall bladder and closure of the cystic duct. It is typically performed laparoscopically and will need intraoperative imaging to demonstrate the integrity and patency of the biliary vessels. This is performed by catheterizing the cystic duct and injecting a contrast agent through it, a procedure known as a 'cholangiogram'.

Patient position

- Supine, on a radio-lucent table, with the upper abdomen away from the centre column of the table
- The patient may be angled head up or down during the case as needed

C-arm approach

- At 90° to the patient's midline from the left side, centring over the right upper quadrant

Key imaging

- *AP view of gall bladder pre-contrast*
- *AP view demonstrating contrast flow from cystic duct to duodenum*

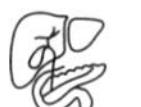

- *AP view demonstrating contrast in left and right hepatic ducts*

Procedure

- The patient is cleaned and draped, and a port is introduced through the umbilicus. Further ports are then introduced to allow access to the gall bladder.

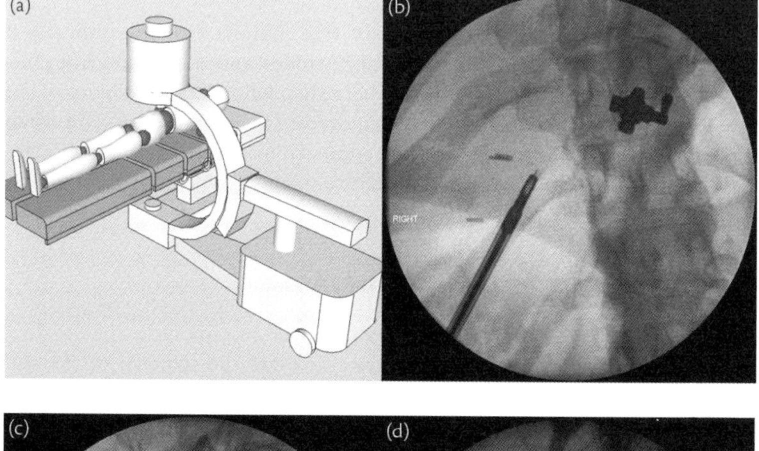

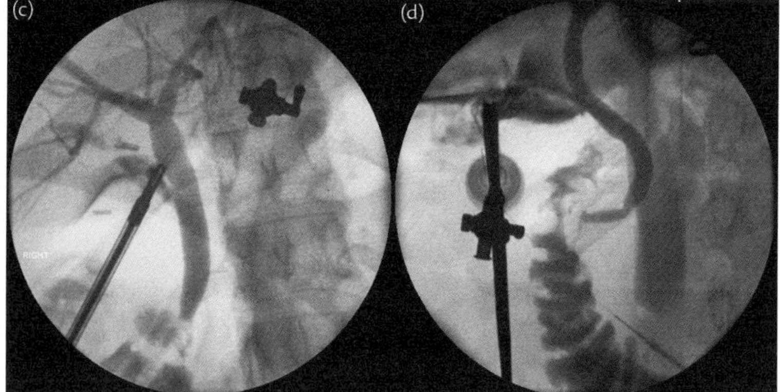

Figure 19.1 Laparoscopic cholangiogram. (a) C-arm approach. Table may be titled head up or down to assist contrast flow to inferior or superior biliary tree, respectively. (b) Anteroposterior (AP) view of catheter in cystic duct. (c) AP view of superior biliary tree. (d) AP of inferior biliary tree showing flow into duodenum.

(b), (c), and (d) Reproduced courtesy of Radiology Department, Leeds Teaching Hospitals NHS Trust, UK.

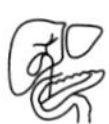

- The cystic duct is located and separated from the surrounding structures. The gall bladder is clamped off as it joins the cystic duct. A catheter is then fed into an opening made on the duct, and secured in place (Figure 19.1).
- The C-arm is draped over the receptor head and brought in from the left side of the patient, so that it is centred over the upper right quadrant. *It is important at this point to avoid striking any of the ports with the receptor head.*
- The position of the C-arm should be checked by taking an image to ensure that the catheter is in the centre of the image. *This image should be saved as a pre-contrast image. Pulsed exposure settings will lower the radiation dose to the patient and theatre staff, but will blur the movement of structures, which may prevent visualization of small stones or leaks of contrast, and as such should be used sparingly.* Once the centring of the C-arm is satisfactory, the cholangiogram may be performed.
- *Contrast is injected down the catheter into the cystic duct, and live screening is used to demonstrate the flow of contrast into the duodenum.* The full lengths of the cystic and common hepatic ducts should be demonstrated in order to identify any leaks or occlusions, as well as the flow of contrast into the duodenum. These images should be saved.
- The table may then be tilted head down, and more contrast injected to demonstrate the superior biliary tree, including the hepatic ducts. *These too should be visualized (by moving the C-arm superiorly), and the images saved.* Once these images are satisfactory, the C-arm can be withdrawn.
- *The pre- and post-contrast images demonstrating the whole of the biliary tree should be sent to the picture archiving and communication system (PACS) along with the dose information.*

19.2 **Endoscopic retrograde cholangiopancreatogram (ERCP)**

Blockages within the biliary system such as stones or strictures can often be treated without removing the gall bladder. The biliary tree can be accessed endoscopically via the sphincter of Oddi within the duodenum. By this route, contrast dye can be injected into the biliary tree to demonstrate it under fluoroscopy, and any occlusions can be identified (cholangiopancreatogram). Once located, strictures can be opened via balloons or stents, and stones can be removed without the need to pierce the abdomen. This reduces the risks of bleeding and infection than with laparoscopic surgery.

Patient position

- Prone or prone decubitus, with right side raised on a radio-lucent table, and the head supported to the right side

C-arm approach

- From the left side of the table, centred over the patient's right upper quadrant

Key imaging

- *PA view of the duodenum to show endoscope and catheter in position*
- *Pre-contrast PA view of the biliary tree*
- *PA screening of liver and biliary tree to show guidewire position*
- *Post-contrast cholangiopancreatogram showing the whole biliary tree and pancreatic duct*
- *PA screening of the biliary tree to show guidewire and surgical hardware*
- *Post-intervention cholangiopancreatogram showing the whole biliary tree and pancreatic duct*

Procedure

- The patient is positioned and sedated, and a mouthpiece inserted. An endoscope is inserted through the mouth and stomach into the duodenum
- The papilla is located and a cannula is fed into it. A guidewire is fed through the cannula into the biliary tree. *Live screening will be required to show the path of the wire and check whether it is in the correct region* (Figure 19.2).
- Contrast may be injected to demonstrate the biliary tree and any strictures or blockages within it. *PA imaging will be required to demonstrate the biliary tree.*
- *Further live screening will be required as any instruments (balloons, cages) are passed over the guidewire to the required areas/occlusions.*
- Once the occlusions have been removed or the stent placed, another image showing the whole of the biliary tree and drainage into the duodenum is required.
- *The pre- and post-contrast images demonstrating the whole of the biliary tree should be sent to the PACS along with the dose information.*

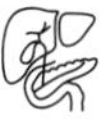

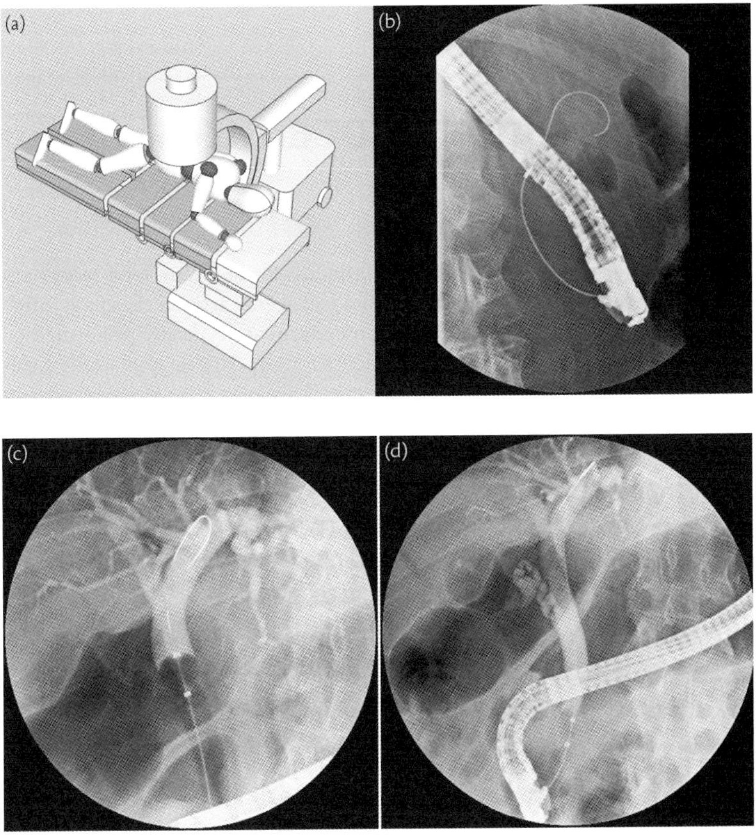

Figure 19.2 Endoscopic retrograde cholangiopancreatogram. (a) Prone decubitus positioning. (b) Resulting image showing endoscope and guidewire in stomach. (c) Post-contrast image of biliary tree with balloon inflated (white markers on wire). (d) Post-contrast image of biliary tree down to common bile duct/duodenum.

(b), (c), and (d) Reproduced courtesy of Radiology Department, Leeds Teaching Hospitals NHS Trust, UK.

References

Cotton, P. B. and Williams, C. B. *Practical Gastrointestinal Endoscopy: The Fundamentals* (Hoboken, 2011).

20

Pain clinic procedures

One of the most commonly offered treatments for medium–long-term back pain is targeted injections of pharmacological agents around the spine (often known as 'injection therapy'). These procedures are typically performed on an outpatient basis, with less requirements for anaesthesia and sterile fields than the more invasive surgical procedures. They may be performed as diagnostic tests, or to give either short- or long-term relief from pain symptoms associated with the spine. Such procedures are also becoming widespread in cases where the symptomatic nerves are damaged or destroyed with heat, cold, lasers, or chemical agents.

Many of these procedures require imaging guidance to correctly target the intended structures around the spine that may be the cause of the symptoms. Typically, these are performed either with a C-arm system or under CT guidance. These procedures are already widely available, and are likely to become even more prevalent in the future as the incidences and effects of chronic back pain rise. As such, it is important for radiographers to be aware of these procedures and the required techniques to correctly perform them. Only procedures performed under C-arm control will be covered here (Silbergleit et al. 2001; Staal et al. 2008).

20.1 Facet joint injections

The facet joints are paired (left and right-sided) articulation points formed by the superior and inferior articular processes of the vertebrae. They allow movement between vertebrae while preventing over-rotation or anterior slippage. Pathology or degenerative changes of the joint can cause pain and restriction of movement. However, as there are many structures around the spine that can cause similar symptoms, a selective intervention at the appropriate facet joint can be performed to either diagnose the cause of symptoms or offer relief from them.

This procedure consists of an injection of medications into the facet joints between vertebrae to numb the surrounding nerve endings. Performed aseptically under imaging control, the procedure involves locating the

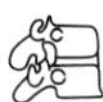

joint(s) under investigation, numbing the surrounding tissues with local anaesthetics, and advancing a spinal needle through the skin so that the tip is within the joint capsule. Linear collimation parallel to the spine can help reduce patient dose and scatter, improving image clarity. The joint is then injected with either diagnostic or therapeutic agents. For therapeutic procedures, the joint is injected with a mixture of local anaesthetics and steroids to block pain signals from the joint. For diagnostic injections, shorter-acting anaesthetics may be used (to see if they give temporary relief from facet pain), or saline/contrast can be injected to distend the joint in an effort to reproduce facet symptoms.

Lumbar facet

- The patient is positioned prone on a radio-lucent table. A pillow or other radio-lucent support may be placed under the abdomen, to reduce lumbar lordosis and help open up the facet joints. The skin surrounding the lumbar spine is cleaned with sterilizing prep and draped.
- The C-arm is brought in at the AP position from the opposite side to the doctor performing the procedure, centred over the spine at roughly the level under investigation. *As the doctors will require access to the patient's back during the procedure, the receptor should be raised high enough to allow them to adjust the positioning of the needles.*
- *Screening may often be performed in the AP position to locate the level of the facet joints under investigation, and this area can then be marked with a sterile marker.* The C-arm can then be rotated to an oblique position (around 15–30°), with the receptor towards the side under investigation. This angle can vary considerably between patients, and adjustments to the angle may hence be required until the joint is clearly demonstrated (Figure 20.1).
- The facets of the upper lumbar spine are typically demonstrated at a less oblique angle than those of the lower vertebrae. Alternatively, the C-arm can be kept in the AP position, and the patient can roll to an oblique position, with the side under investigation facing up towards the receptor head. Supports under the patient (e.g. a pillow) will help him or her maintain this position.
- *The joint to be injected will then be located and the entry point for the needle identified.* The joint itself should be seen in profile (between the head/ear of the 'scotty dog' on the inferior vertebrae and the front leg on the superior one).
- The doctor performing the procedure will numb the area with local anaesthetics before inserting the spinal needle towards the joint. The

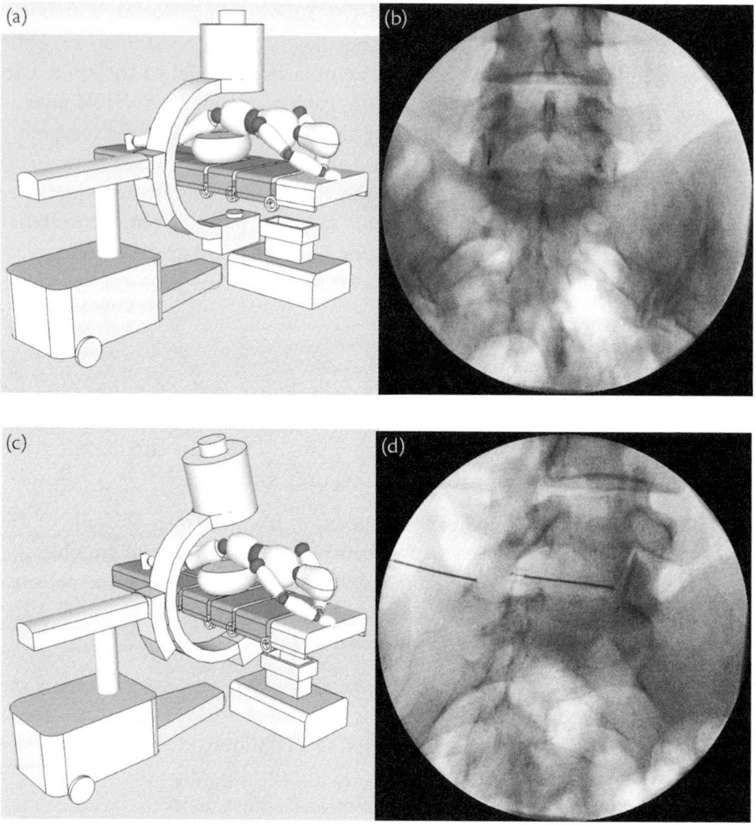

Figure 20.1 Lumbar facet joint injection. (a) Anteroposterior view of lumbar spine positioning. (b) Resulting image showing bilateral needles at L5–S1 level. (c) Oblique view of lumbar spine to demonstrate facet joints. (d) Resulting image. Note 'scotty dog' appearance.

(b) and (d) Reproduced courtesy of Radiology Department, Leeds Teaching Hospitals NHS Trust, UK.

depth of the needle in relation to the joint is checked by the doctor feeling for resistance as the needle progresses. *However, if there is any uncertainty about the position of the needle tip, a less rotated view can be performed (once the original oblique appears satisfactory) to demonstrate the depth of the needle in relation to the vertebrae.*

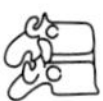

- Alternatively, live screening can be used as the C-arm is rotated slowly back to the AP position. *A small amount of iodinated contrast can also be injected to demonstrate the joint.*
- Once the correct needle position is confirmed, the medications (typically a mix of local anaesthetics and steroids) are injected into the joint, and the needle is removed. *Images demonstrating the needle in position should be saved and archived.* Further injections may take place on the opposite side and at different spinal levels.

Thoracic facet

- Thoracic facet injections are performed in a similar manner to lumbar facet injections. The patient is positioned prone on a radio-lucent table, with the C-arm brought in opposite from where the doctor will be working. However, the facet joints are angled more laterally than in the lumbar spine, and so the C-arm will need to be angled more to demonstrate them in profile for the oblique views.
- *A lateral view may also be used to demonstrate the depth of the needle, performed by rotating the C-arm under the table to horizontal.* Contrast injections into the joint may also be used to highlight the joint against the ribs and other bony structures around the facet.
- *Pre- and post-contrast images should be saved and archived to the picture archiving and communication system (PACS) along with the dose information.*

Cervical facet

- *For cervical facet joints, the C-arm may be positioned to demonstrate the spine in a true lateral position.* The patient may be positioned on his or her side (with the affected side raised), or in a sitting position with the head supported on a rest.
- Alternatively, some doctors will prefer an anterior oblique position, where the patient is positioned supine and then turned 45°, so that the affected side is raised. *Whichever position is used, the patient should drop his or her shoulders as far as possible to better demonstrate the inferior cervical vertebrae, and supports should be used to avoid any lateral flexion of the neck.*
- The patient's neck may be flexed anteriorly to help open the joints. If the patient is positioned on his or her side (with the C-arm in the undercouch position), oblique views can be performed if needed by rotating the C-arm. Similarly, if they are in the oblique position, rotation of the C-arm can give a true lateral view.

- *Once the C-arm is positioned to demonstrate the spine, collimation can be used to avoid irradiation of the orbits.* Screening will be used to locate the level of the facet joint under investigation before the area around it is numbed with local anaesthetics.
- The spinal needle is then inserted upwards towards the joint. *Screening will be used to check the position of the needle as it is advanced, before the medications are injected.* AP views may also be obtained to check the needle position. *Images demonstrating the needle in position (either before or after the injection) should be saved and archived to the PACS along with the dose information.*

20.2 Nerve root injections

The nerve roots are paired segments of nerve fibre bundles that branch away from the spinal cord through the intervertebral foramina. Impingement of the root around the foramen (e.g. by disk herniation or stenosis of the foramen) can cause pain that radiates away from the spine. In such cases, a selective nerve root injection may be performed to either identify the source of pain or reduce symptoms. These are performed in a manner similar to facet joint injections, consisting of a targeted injection of medications such as local anaesthetics or steroids into a region of anatomy that is believed to be the source of pain. However, this procedure places the medication around the outside of the nerve that is being targeted, rather than within a joint. It is very important during such procedures to avoid any damage to the nerve itself with the needle tip, and as such accurate positioning of the needle under imaging control is required.

Lumbar nerve root

- The patient is positioned prone on a radio-lucent table, and may then be turned so that the affected side is raised, and supported with a pillow or other radio-lucent item underneath the affected side. The skin surrounding the lumbar spine is cleaned with sterilizing prep and draped.
- The C-arm is brought in at the AP position from the opposite side to the doctor performing the procedure, centred over the spine at roughly the level under investigation. *As the doctors will require access to the patient's back during the procedure, the receptor should be raised high enough to allow them to adjust the positioning of the needles.*
- *Screening may often be performed in the AP position to locate the level of the intervertebral foramina under investigation, and this area can then be marked with a sterile marker.*

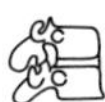

- The needle is then slowly advanced underneath the pedicles to the nerve root. *AP and lateral views will be required to check the position of the needle tip in relation to the anatomy.* Once the needle tip appears in the correct position, the most recent views should be saved.
- *Contrast can then be injected to highlight the anatomy around the needle tip. This will need to be checked in AP view, which should also be saved as a post-contrast image.* Once the root is visualized with the contrast, the required medications are injected around it. Further injections may then take place on the opposite side and at different spinal levels.
- *The saved pre- and post-contrast images demonstrating each nerve root injected should then be saved to the PACS along with the dose information.*

20.3 Epidural injections

If more targeted injections do not alleviate symptoms, an epidural can be performed. These are injections of steroids or other therapeutic material into the epidural space, via either the lumbar spine or sacrum. Image guidance is required for these procedures to ensure that the therapeutic agents are injected into the correct region. This can be checked by visualizing the needle tip in relation to the spinal anatomy and by injecting the suitable contrast medium into the epidural space (Fritz et al. 2007).

Lumbar epidural

- The patient is positioned prone, and the area over the lumbar spine is cleaned and draped. The C-arm is brought in at 90° from the patient's midline, from the side opposite to the surgeon, so that the receptor head is centred over the patient's lumbar spine.
- *The position for insertion of the needle may be checked by placing the tip of a spinal needle over the patient's spine and then performing an AP image.* Linear collimation parallel to the lumbar spine can reduce radiation dose to the patient and surgeon while performing this view.
- Once the entry point is satisfactory, the needle is slowly advanced into the epidural space. The position of the needle tip in relation to the epidural space is checked by feeling for a change of resistance in the syringe. As such, imaging is not generally required for this part, and the C-arm may be withdrawn.
- *Once the needle is advanced into the epidural space, the position may be checked under X-ray.* The C-arm is brought back in with the receptor head over

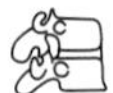

the needle. *Contrast may also be injected to outline the epidural space, and, if this is performed, pre- and post-contrast images should be saved.*

- Once the required area is demonstrated with contrast, therapeutic agents are injected through the needle into the required area. Another AP view may be required at this point to demonstrate the dilution of contrast by the therapeutic agents. This image should also be saved. *The C-arm can then be withdrawn, and all saved images should be sent to the PACS along with the dose report.*

Caudal epidural

- The patient is positioned prone, and the region around the sacrum is cleaned and draped. The C-arm is brought in at 90° from the patient's midline from the opposite side to the surgeon, so that the receptor head is centred over the patient's sacrum.
- The location for insertion of the spinal needle is found by the surgeon palpating along the length of the sacrum. *The position may also be checked by placing the tip of a spinal needle over the patient's sacrum and then performing an AP image.* Once the insertion point is confirmed, the AP image should be saved, and the needle inserted and advanced towards the sacral canal (Figure 20.2).

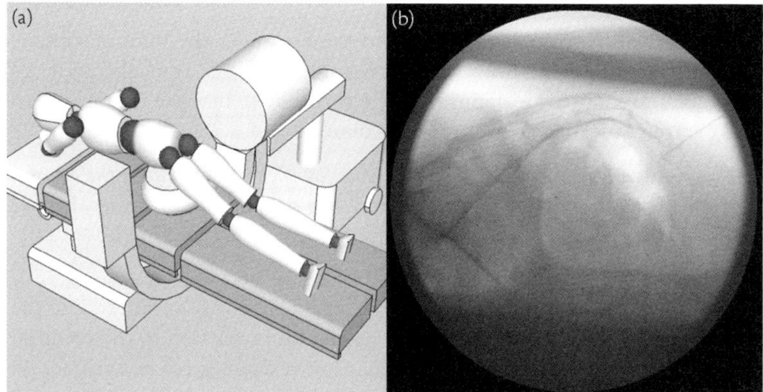

Figure 20.2 Caudal/sacral epidural. (a) Lateral positioning for epidural (caudal) injection. (b) Resulting lateral image. Note: collimation used to better demonstrate sacrum.

(b) Reproduced courtesy of Radiology Department, Leeds Teaching Hospitals NHS Trust, UK.

 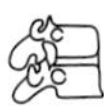

- *The C-arm is now rotated under-table to give a lateral view of the patients' sacrum. Linear collimation may be used parallel to the sacrum to reduce scatter and improve image quality, as well as to reduce radiation dose to the patient and team.* Electronic magnification may also be of use to better visualize the needle within the canal.
- *The needle is slowly advanced, and its depth checked under lateral view.* An AP view may also be required. *Once the needle tip appears in place, the lateral view should be saved before contrast is injected into the sacral canal.* The needle position is then checked by ensuring no cerebrospinal fluid is flowing back into the syringe. *Once contrast has been injected, another image may be taken to demonstrate the position of the needle tip and flow of contrast. This image should also be saved.*
- Once the required area is demonstrated with contrast, therapeutic agents are injected through the needle into the required area. *Another lateral view may be required at this point to demonstrate the dilution of contrast by the therapeutic agents.* This image should also be saved. *The C-arm can then be withdrawn, and all saved images should be sent to the PACS along with the dose report.*

References

Fritz, J., Niemeyer, T., Clasen, S., Wiskirchen, J., Tepe, G., Kastler, B., Nägele, T., König, C., Claussen, C., and Pereira, P. 'Management of Chronic Low Back Pain: Rationales, Principles, and Targets of Imaging-guided Spinal Injections', *Radiographics*, 27 (2007), 1751–1771.

Silbergleit, R., Mehta, B., Sanders, W., and Talati, S. 'Imaging-Guided Injection Techniques with Fluoroscopy and CT for Spinal Pain Management', *Radiographics*, 21 (2001), 927–942.

Staal, J. B., de Bie, R., de Vet, H. C. W., Hildebrandt, J., and Nelemans, P. 'Injection Therapy for Subacute and Chronic Low-back Pain', *Cochrane Database of Systematic Reviews*, 3 (2008), Art. No.: CD001824. doi: 10.1002/14651858.CD001824.pub3.

Index

Figures are indicated by an italic *f* following the page number.